Lu K'uan Yu (Charles Luk) was born in Canton in 1898. He was a lay disciple of two famous Ch'an masters and devoted himself to presenting 'as many Chinese Buddhist texts as possible so that Buddhism can be preserved in the West'. He died in 1978.

By the same author

Taoist Yoga

Alchemy and Immortality

LU K'UAN YU

A translation (with introduction and notes) of
The Secrets of Cultivating Essential Nature and Eternal Life
(Hsin Ming Fa Chueh Ming Chik) by the Taoist Master Chao Pi
Ch'en, born 1860

RIDER
LONDON SYDNEY AUCKLAND JOHANNESBURG

1 3 5 7 9 10 8 6 4 2

First published in Great Britain by Rider in 1970
This edition first published in 1996
Rider is an imprint of Ebury Press,
Random House, 20 Vauxhall Bridge Road,
London SW1V 2SA

Random House Australia (Pty) Limited
20 Alfred Street, Milsons Point, Sydney,
New South Wales 2061, Australia

Random House New Zealand Limited
18 Poland Road, Glenfield,
Auckland 10, New Zealand

Random House South Africa (Pty) Limited
PO Box 337, Bergvlei 2012, South Africa

Random House UK Limited Reg. No. 954009

Papers used by Rider Books are natural, recyclable products made
from wood grown in sustainable forests. In addition, the paper in this
book is recycled

Typeset by SX Composing DTP, Rayleigh, Essex
Printed by Guernsey Press Ltd

A CIP catalogue record for this book is available from the
British Library

ISBN 0-7126-1725-6

This book is reverently dedicated to my godfather, the Deity Pe Ti, ruler of the Northern Heaven, who has helpfully guided me in my translation of Taoist Scriptures herein presented

CONTENTS

ILLUSTRATIONS

PREFACE

After the publication of our fourth book, *The Secrets of Chinese Meditation,* and its Italian and German translations,[1] we have been delighted to hear from Western readers who have practised Indian yoga and are also interested in studying its Chinese equivalent. But only three chapters of that volume deal with Taoist meditation for the improvement of health, so that for lack of space we were unable to deal fully with Taoist yoga, which includes spiritual alchemy and aims at the total defeat of mortality.

This presentation is a translation of *The Secrets of Cultivation of Essential Nature and Eternal Life,* written by the Taoist master Chao Pi Ch'en (born 1860) and containing a comprehensive exposition of Taoist yoga with instructions by the ancients which can be studied and practised by modern students. It consists of sixteen chapters which teach how to train in spiritual alchemy from the beginning to the end in order to leap over the mortal to the undying divine state.

[1] *The Secrets of Chinese Meditation,* Rider & Co., London; *I Segreti della Meditazione Cinese,* Ubaldini Editore, Rome; and *Geheimnisse der chinesischen Meditation,* Rascher Verlag, Zürich and Stuttgart. Its French translation is being undertaken by a well known publisher in Paris.

Taoist scriptures are full of technical terms which seem very obscure and unintelligible even to students in China, for the authors did not intend to make the texts accessible to people of low spirituality or of questionable character, or to unbelievers and blasphemers. Instead of translating them literally we have rendered them in simple English in order to avoid confusion. For instance, *lead* and *mercury* are translated by *vitality* and *spirit,* for which they stand, so as to make the text more clear for the average reader. We have, however, kept some terms for which there are no English equivalents with accompanying explanations or footnotes so that Western readers will appreciate that we too encountered great difficulty when we began to study these Taoist texts.

Taoist alchemy forsakes the worldly way of life by preventing the generative force which produces the generative fluid from following its ordinary course which satisfies sexual desire and procreates offspring. As soon as this force moves to find its usual outlet, it is turned back and then driven by the inner fire, kindled by regulated breathing, into the microcosmic orbit for sublimation. This orbit begins at the base of the spine, called the first gate (wei lu), rising in the backbone to the second gate between the kidneys (chia chi), and then to the back of the head, called the third gate (yu ch'en), before reaching the brain (ni wan). It then descends down the face, chest and abdomen to return to where it rose and so completes a full circuit.

By regulated breathing is meant deep breathing that reaches the lower abdomen to arouse the inner fire and then bring pressure on the generative force already held there forcing both fire and generative force to rise in the channel of control in the spine to the head. This is followed by an out breathing which relaxes the lower abdomen so that the fire and generative force that have risen to the head sink in the channel of function in the front of the body to form a full rotation in the microcosmic orbit. These continued ascents and descents cleanse and purify the generative force which is then held in the lower tan t'ien under the navel so that it can be transmuted into vitality.

The microcosmic orbit has four cardinal points: at the root of the penis where the generative force is gathered, at the top of the head, and at the two points between them in the spine and in the front of the body where the generative force is cleansed and purified during the microcosmic orbiting.

While putting the generative force into orbit it is of paramount importance to locate the original cavity of spirit in the brain which is precisely where a light manifests in the head when the practiser succeeds in concentrating his seeing effectively on the central spot between and behind the eyes. If this is not done the radiant inner fire rising to the head during the microcosmic orbiting may be mistaken for that light and wrongly driven into a minor psychic centre in the head from which it will be very difficult to dislodge it. Many untutored and inexperienced practisers make this mistake which hinders the process of alchemy.

When the generative force moves to obey its worldly inclination, the purpose of regulating the breathing is to draw the force up to the lower tan t'ien cavity under the navel so as to hold it there and transmute it into an alchemical agent which is transformed into vitality in the solar plexus. Thus the lower tan t'ien in the lower abdomen plays the role of a burning stove supporting a cauldron which contains the generative force ready for subsequent ascension to the solar plexus.

After being purified the generative force is carried in the microcosmic orbit to the solar plexus, called the middle tan t'ien, which becomes the middle cauldron and is scorched by the burning stove in the lower tan t'ien under the navel. It is in the solar plexus that the generative force (now the alchemical agent) is transmuted into vitality which rises to the brain (ni wan) where the vital breath, hitherto hidden and dormant, will be stirred by well regulated breathing which will prevent it from dispersing. The precious cauldron has now manifested in the brain (ni wan) whereas the burning stove remains in the lower tan t'ien under the navel.

So while the stove remains in the lower abdomen during the whole process of alchemy, the cauldron changes place rising from the lower tan t'ien under the navel to the middle tan t'ien or solar plexus, and finally to the upper tan t'ien in the brain where it is called the precious cauldron. In other words, the lower tan t'ien plays the role of primary cauldron which contains the generative force at the start of the process of alchemy. When the generative force is cleansed and purified during the microcosmic orbiting and becomes the alchemical agent, it rises to the solar plexus which then plays the role of the middle cauldron in which the generative force is transmuted into vitality. When vitality is purified it rises to the ni wan or brain which then becomes the precious cauldron in which vitality is transmuted into spirit. Thus the lower, middle and upper tan t'ien successively become the cauldron which means the cavity or psychic centre in which transmutation actually takes place.

The practiser thus 'lays the foundation' by gathering the microcosmic outer alchemical agent[2] to restore the generative force that has dispersed and so to invigorate the brain. The method consists of deep and regulated breathing to raise the

---

[2]See Chapter 2, *figure 1*, for detailed explanation of inhalation and exhalation of outer air to kindle the inner fire to cleanse and purity the generative force during the microcosmic orbiting. The microcosmic outer alchemical agent is so called because it is produced by means of fresh air breathed in and out to transmute the generative force into vitality.

inner fire in the channel of control to the brain thirty-six times and thence lower it in the channel of function in the front of the body twenty-four times, the numbers thirty-six and twenty-four being positive and negative numbers in Taoist yoga. Each rotation is completed in a full in-and-out breath during which spirit and vitality move and halt together in the juxtaposed orbits of the earth (the body) and heaven (the head), spirit being set in motion by the movements of the eyes and vitality by the combined action of the vital and generative forces already gathered. This is how to gather the outer alchemical agent to free the body from all ailments.

The microcosmic inner alchemical agent[3] is now gathered by rolling the eyes from left to right in conjunction with the microcosmic fire that passes through sublimating phases at the four cardinal points of the microcosmic orbit. This process is called the 'inner copulation' of the positive and negative principles. It means that vitality, driven by ventilation (breathing) and (inner) fire, soars up and down so that the vital breath in the brain unites with the nervous system, causing spirit to develop and its bright light to manifest; this is commonly called the preparation of the 'golden elixir'. This bright light is the mysterious gate (hsuan kuan) which is indescribable and from which spirit emerges for the breakthrough.

The eyes are positive, whereas the rest of the body is negative. Therefore, when the outer alchemical agent has been gathered, it is necessary to roll the eyes to unite the positive with the negative principles in order to develop spirit in the bright light that emerges from the original cavity of spirit between and behind the eyes. This bright light shows the exact position of that cavity and should not be confounded with the

---

[3]See Chapter 6, *figure 5*, for detailed explanation of the microcosmic inner alchemical agent which is so called because it is produced by vital breath in the body, used to transmute vitality into spirit.

luminous inner fire that rises to the head during the microcosmic orbiting as we have said earlier. In Taoist yoga the negative vitality is represented by the dragon and the positive vitality by the tiger, while their 'copulation' brings into manifestation the original spirit in its bright light.

When original or prenatal spirit manifests thus, it should be driven into the lower tan t'ien centre under the navel to fix it there. This centre has outer and inner cells: the outer cell is the source of the positive and negative principles, the abode of vital breath, the source of foetal breathing and the mechanism of in and out breathing; and the inner cell is where the immortal foetus is created and the vital breath stays; it is the house of serenity. When the vital breath, moving up and down in the thrusting channel (see *figure* 8, page 141) does not rise above the heart (the house of fire) and drop below the lower abdomen (the house of water) it will slip into this cavity under the navel, causing the sudden manifestation of true serenity.

The practiser should now concentrate on the lower tan t'ien cavity under the navel until vitality vibrates there, then lift it to the heart (the seat of fire) and lower it to the lower abdomen (the seat of water) with continued ascents and descents in the thrusting channel until suddenly it slips into that cavity; this is called 're-entry into the foetus for further creativity' and is the outcome of linking the heart (fire) with the lower abdomen (water). Spirit which has been fixed there will be enveloped by vitality until both unite into a whole, called the immortal foetus in the state of complete serenity.

When this state is reached it is necessary to practise immortal breathing through the heel channel starting from the heels and the trunk channel from the lower abdomen to the brain (see *figure* 7 page 105), in order to achieve the self-turning of the wheel of the law, called the macrocosmic orbit or the free circulation of vital breathing through the former and down through the latter channel to restore the profound foetal breathing which wipes out all postnatal conditions so that pre-natal vitality can be transmuted into a bright pearl that illumi-nates the brain. This means that after the sublimation of the generative force, vitality and spirit, they gather in the brain where, under constant pressure from prenatal vitality and spirit, they will in time produce an ambrosia. This ambrosia (which is not to be confused with the golden elixir) then pro-duces and nurtures the immortal seed in the lower tan t'ien cavity under the navel, where it radiates, lighting up the heart. This light reveals the formation of the immortal seed when all breathing appears to cease and pulses seem to stop beating in the condition of complete serenity.

The cultivation of immortality does not go beyond spirit and vitality. Spirit leads to the realisation of essential nature and vitality to eternal life. When the generative force is full and rises to unite with essential nature, the white light of vitality manifests; it is like moonlight and its fullness is equivalent to one half of a whole. When vitality is full and descends to unite with eternal life, the golden light manifests; it is reddish yellow and its fullness is equivalent to the other half. The union of these two lights produces that whole which is the immortal seed.

After the immortal seed has returned to its source in the lower abdomen, a pointed concentration on it will, in time, cause a golden light to appear in the white light between the eyebrows. This is the embryo of the immortal seed produced by the union of the generative force, vitality and spirit into one whole. These two lights are like the male and female organs of a flower, the union of which will bear fruit.

At the manifestation of this positive light, which is the union of the two lights, the practiser should stop the fire and concentrate in the head the vital breaths in the heart, stomach, liver, lungs and lower abdomen to produce the macrocosmic alchemical agent which should be gathered to achieve the final breakthrough, thereby leaping over the worldly to the saintly state, and so leaving the state of serenity to appear in countless transformation bodies.

When this state is reached the practiser should unite the two vitalities of nature and life to help spirit form the immortal foetus. It is only after flying snow and falling flowers have been seen by the practiser that spirit emerges from the foetus to become immortal. He should now 'stir the thought' of leaping into the great emptiness which will open the heavenly gate at the top of the head so that spirit can leave the human body to appear in countless bodies in space.

In the text 'prenatal' denotes the positive or spiritual nature originally existing before birth and 'postnatal' means its negative or corrupt counterpart which follows the ordinary way of material life after birth, the former being real and permanent whereas the latter is illusory and transient.

The lower tan t'ien under the navel is also called the cavity or ocean of vitality.

According to Arthur Avalon (Sir John Woodroffe), an authority on Tantric yoga, some modern pundits tend to misplace the psychic centres or cavities in the body. I would urge readers to guard against these arbitrary speculations. When they have made real progress in their practice of Taoist yoga, they will automatically know where in the body these psychic centres really are, for the latter usually feel warm when the inner fire passes through them during its circulation in the microcosmic orbit. It is harmful to pinpoint places in the body, the very idea of which should be relinquished since it hinders the course of the inner fire and of vitality.

Like Western authors who use numbers and letters of the alphabet to indicate successive chapters of a book and different parts of a diagram, their Chinese counterparts use the ten Heavenly Stems (chia, i, ping, ting, wu, chi, keng, hsin, jen, kuei) to mark successive parts of their books and the twelve Earthly Branches (tzu, ch'ou, yin, mao, ch'en, szu, wu, wei, shen, yu, shu, hai) to show various parts of their illustrations. For instance, the twelve divisions of the microcosmic orbit are indicated by twelve Chinese characters which are the above twelve Earthly Branches in the original diagrams which are reproduced in this book with the first twelve letters of the alphabet (A to L) for the convenience of Western readers. The ten Heavenly Stems are used with the twelve Earthly Branches to form a cycle to indicate the hours, days, months and years in the Chinese almanac. They are also employed in medical science, astronomy, astrology, physiognomy, palmistry, etc.

All brackets are mine and are added to make the ancient texts more clear.

Hongkong   LU K'UAN YU

1

FIXING SPIRIT IN ITS ORIGINAL CAVITY

My masters Liao Jan and Liao K'ung once said: 'When beginning to cultivate (essential) nature and (eternal) life, it is necessary first to develop nature.' Before sitting in meditation, it is important to put an end to all rising thoughts and to loosen garments and belt to relax the body and avoid interfering with the free circulation of blood. After sitting the body should be (senseless) like a log and the heart (mind) unstirred like cold ashes. The eyes should look down and fix on the tip of the nose; they should not be shut completely to avoid dullness and confusion; neither should they be wide open to prevent spirit from wandering outside. They should be fixed on the tip of the nose with one's attention concentrated on the spot between them; and in time the light of vitality will manifest. This is the best way to get rid of all thoughts at the start when preparing the elixir of immortality.

When the heart (mind) is settled, one should restrain the faculty of seeing, check that of hearing, touch the palate with the tip of the tongue and regulate the breathing through the nostrils. If breathing is not regulated one will be troubled by gasping or laboured breaths. When breathing is well controlled, one will forget all about the body and heart (mind).

Thus stripped of feelings and passions one will look like a stupid man.

The left leg should be placed outside and close to the right one; this means the positive embracing the negative.[1] The thumb of the left hand should touch its middle finger and the right hand should be placed under it (palm upward) with its thumb bent over the left palm; this means the negative embracing the positive. This is what the ancients meant by forming a circuit of eight psychic channels. The Taoist scriptures say: 'The linking of the four limbs shuts the four gates so that the centre can be held on to.'

Question I have read Taoist books which all urge the development of the light in the original cavity or centre of spirit (tsu ch'iao, in the centre of the brain between and behind the eyes) at the start of practice but I do not see why. All Taoist schools regard this as the aim of the cultivation of (essential) nature without giving details. Will you please tell me where true nature actually manifests?

Answer (The tsu ch'iao cavity in) the centre of the brain branches out into two minor channels on its left and right; the left one stands for t'ai chi (supreme ultimate) and the right one for ch'ung ling (immaterial spirit); they are linked with the t'ien ku (heavenly valley) centre above them and the yung chuan (bubbling spring) centres in the soles of the feet after running through the heart in the chest.

The Tan Ching says: 'Nature is (in) the heart and manifests through the eyes; life is (in) the lower abdomen and manifests through the genital organ.'

(Essential) nature is spiritual vitality in the heart that manifests through the two channels from the centre of the

[1]This posture will help some Westerners who cannot sit with crossed legs.

brain. So when seeing is concentrated on the spot between the eyes, the light of (essential) nature manifests and will, after a long training, unite with (eternal) life to become one whole. This union is called seeing the void that is not empty and he who is not awakened to this union will achieve nothing in his practice.

Question When I was taught meditation I was urged to empty my heart (the house of fire) of all thoughts, set my mind on cultivating (essential) nature and open my eyes to contemplate the void to accord with the correct way; will you please explain all this to me?

Answer Seeing the void as not empty is right and seeing the void as empty is wrong, for failure to return to the (tsu ch'iao) centre (which is not empty) prevents the light of vitality from manifesting. Under the heart and above the genital organ is an empty space where spiritual vitality manifests to form a cavity. When spirit and vitality return to this cavity, spiritual vitality will soar up to form a circle (of light) which is not void. Voidness which does not radiate is relative but voidness which radiates is absolute. Absolute voidness is not empty like relative voidness. Voidness that is not empty is spiritual light which is spirit-vitality that springs from the yellow hall centre (huang ting or middle tan t'ien, in the solar plexus).

My master Liao K'ung said: 'When the golden mechanism (of alchemy) begins to move and gives out flashes of light that hall of voidness (hsu shih, i.e. the heart devoid of feelings and passions) will be illuminated by a white light which reveals the mysterious gate (hsuan kuan)[2], the presence of which does not mean emptiness.

Man lives and dies because of this immaterial spirit-

[2]Mysterious entrance to immortality.

vitality; he lives when it is present and dies when it scatters. Hence it is said: 'Spirit without vitality does not make a man live; and vitality without spirit does not cause him to die.' Prenatal spirit in the heart is nature and prenatal vitality in the lower abdomen is life; only when spirit and vitality unite can real achievement be made.

Question Will you please explain the saying: 'If one reaches the original cavity of spirit (tsu ch'iao, in the centre of the brain between and behind the eyes) one will find the source of immortal breath.'?

Answer Worldly men who discover the original cavity of spirit are very rare indeed. It is under heaven (the top of the head), above the earth (the lower abdomen), west of the sun (the left eye) and east of the moon (the right eye). Behind the mysterious gate (hsuan kuan) and before the spirit of the valley (ku shen) is true nature (chen hsin) which is the source of true breath (chen hsi). Although this true breath is linked with postnatal (ordinary) breathing, the latter coming in-and-out through the mouth and nostrils, cannot reach the original cavity of spirit to return to the source. The immortal breath that comes from inner (vital) fourfold breathing[3] and not through the nose and mouth), can then return to the source.

In your quest for immortal breath, you should regulate postnatal (ordinary) breathing in order to find its source. This immortal breath is hidden in the original cavity of spirit and is genial and will not scatter away when postnatal (ordinary) breathing is well regulated. Hence my master Liao Jen said: 'When vitality returns to the original ocean (its source) life becomes boundless.'

[3]A full fourfold breathing consists of in and out breaths with corresponding ascent and descent of vitality in the microcosmic orbit.

Question Will you please give me the exact position of the original cavity of spirit?

Answer It is (in the centre of the brain behind) the spot between the eyes. Lao Tsu called it 'the gateway to heaven and earth'; hence he urged people to concentrate on the centre in order to realise the oneness (of all things). In this centre is a pearl of the size of a grain of rice), which is the centre between heaven and earth in the human body (i.e. the microcosm); it is the cavity of prenatal vitality. To know where it lies is not enough, for it does not include the wondrous light of (essential) nature which is symbolised by a circle which Confucius called virtuous perfection (jen); the Book of Change calls it the ultimateless (wu chi), the Buddha perfect knowledge (yuan ming) and the Taoists the elixir of immortality or spiritual light; which all point to the prenatal One True Vitality. He who knows this cavity can prepare the elixir of immortality. Hence it is said: 'When the One is attained, all problems are solved.'

Therefore, during the training both eyes should turn inward to the centre (between and behind them) in order to hold on to this One which should be held in the original cavity of spirit (tsu ch'iao) with neither strain nor relaxation; this is called fixing spirit in its original cavity which should be where (essential) *nature* is cultivated and the root from which (eternal) *life* emerges.

My master Liao Jan said: 'If the original cavity of spirit is overlooked true breath will not stay permanently, spirit will lack a basis for sublimation, the alchemical agent will be incomplete, and the golden elixir cannot be produced.' For this cavity (between and behind the eyes) is the foundation of (spiritual) stability and the centre of all things, having neither outside nor inside, which cannot be held on to by mindfulness and sought by mindlessness, because to be mindful of it is clinging to the visible and to be mindless leads to (relative) voidness. Then what sort of training should be undergone (to realise it)? The correct method consists of closing both eyes to still the heart (mind) so that the tsu ch'iao cavity can be held on to until the light of (essential) nature appears to confirm its effectiveness.

The practiser should close his mouth and touch the palate with the tongue to immobilise spirit and vitality. When thought is right so is the heart between heaven (the head) and earth (the lower abdomen) and when spirit is pure, the supreme ultimate (t'ai chi) will be well understood. If the non-rising of a single thought is achieved this will in time lead to the state of clearness and purity. In the complete voidness (of sense data) and utter stillness, a white light will manifest to light up the empty heart (hsu shih) and the golden mechanism will give out flashes of light. You will then be automatically clear about the heart of heaven and earth.

Question All schools teach their students to close the mouth and touch the palate with the tongue. Some also urge them to lift the tongue to the palate when they breathe out and to lower it when they breathe in; they call the tongue a key. Is this correct?

Answer All this teaches worldly men to behave properly in the earthly way in order to induce them later to seek immortality; this has nothing to do with the quest of (essential) nature and (eternal) life.

These ascents and descents of air serve solely to restore the generative force and to fortify the brain when men grow old. For most people by indulging in passions and sexual pleasures shorten the span of life, thereby injuring the source of vitality. Hence this teaching on preserving the generative force and strengthening the lower abdomen, the aim of which is to conserve the positive principle for rejuvenation.

Therefore, seekers of immortality should begin by practising the method of preserving the generative force by strengthening the lower abdomen.

My master Liao K'ung said: 'The cavity of the Heavenly Pool (t'ien chih hsueh) is in the palate, and since it is linked with the brain above, it lets vitality flow down and drain away; so the tongue is lifted up to support that pool thereby making a bridge for true vitality[4] to come down through the hsuan ying cavity (the mysterious bridle on the channel of function behind the heavenly pool in the palate) to the lower tan t'ien centre (the field of elixir below the navel) where it is held (for alchemical reasons).'

So if the tip of the tongue touches the palate vitality will gather in front of the original cavity of spirit (tsu ch'iao between and behind the eyes, which will easily become the object of contemplation) being always seen by the eyes (when closed and turned back); always heard by the ears (when they listen for it); always felt by the tongue that supports it and always aimed at by thoughts.

Therefore, this original cavity of spirit should be concentrated on whether the practiser walks, stands, sits or reclines. And all of a sudden the heart becomes pure and the spirits high causing vitality to be overwhelming and the body robust. In this utter stillness devoid of thoughts and feelings the practiser will awaken fully to the void that is not empty and to his (essential) nature. When this stage is reached his vitality develops further, his knowledge increases and his spiritual disposition becomes all-pervading. Unexpectedly a spark of

[4]True vitality is vital force which has been purified by the alchemical process.

real positive (principle) appears revealing the mysterious gate (hsuan kuan).

Hence my master Ch'iao Ch'iao said: 'The mysterious gate has no fixed position; its path is the central passage (see *figure* 8; page 141) (formed by the channel P-M that links the centre of the brain with the heart and the thrusting channel M-A) which passes through the huang ting (or yellow hall) centre N (the solar plexus).'

If the tip of the tongue is not pressed against the heavenly pool vitality will not flow into the lower tan t'ien cavity (under the navel) and the prenatal breath will drain away. This is the immortal breath of the immortal man (chen jen).

Question I have just begun to study Taoist meditation and am still unable to distinguish between the right and wrong teaching. Will you please enlighten me?

Answer In your practice it is most important to distinguish between what is right and wrong. The true Tao is prenatal spirit-vitality. Spirit is (essential) nature and vitality is (eternal) life which is the essential generative force. So vitality is inherent in the generative force.

The patriarch Liu said: 'If the original cavity of spirit (between and behind the eyes) is constantly held on to (i.e. concentrated upon) vital force will develop of itself and will beget true vitality which will be linked with (essential) life in the lower tan t'ien centre (under the navel) to produce the golden elixir (chin tan).' The patriarch feared that students might not know the correct method when vitality manifests and so might let it drain away by the genital duct (yang kuan) to create offspring. When the generative force is half-way down the duct, if the practiser has received correct instruction from a competent master, he will be able to turn it back and use it to prepare the elixir of immortality. Thus we know that the generative force tends to flow away. So when the genital organ is aroused and the penis stands during sleep, it is imperative to breathe in and out to gather the alchemical agent.

My elder brother Chao Kuei I said: 'When the generative force is about to flow out, if the mortal gate (sheng szu ch'iao at the root of the penis) is not blocked (by a finger pressed on it) it will leave by that gate, turn liquid and become the generative fluid which will be discharged. This generative force will become semen if it flows out in the worldly way but will change into vitality if it is turned back (and sublimated in the microcosmic orbit).'

So a student meeting his teacher should first ask him about the proper method and inquire whether or not it consists of gathering outside air to turn it into the alchemical agent. If the teacher denies this and says that his method is to turn back the flow of generative force to fortify the body so that it will be restored to its original condition before puberty and cause the penis to cease standing during sleep and to retract, his is the authentic method.

As to the alchemical agent, if the practiser is unmindful of it when gathering it, it is the prenatal microcosmic agent, but if he is mindful of it it will be an illusory agent which leads only to failure.

2

THE MICROCOSMIC CAULDRON AND STOVE

The precious cauldron (yu ting) is a cavity in the centre of the brain (between and behind the eyes) and is the seat of (essential) nature, that is the original cavity of spirit (yuan shen shih or the ancestral cavity, tsu ch'iao); its left and right sides are linked with the pupils of the eyes by two (psychic) channels; and it is also connected with the heart.[1] Hence it is said that essential nature is (in) the heart which manifests through the two eyes.

It is also said that essential nature is in the precious cauldron which originally did not exist. It is only when true vitality develops and unites with essential nature to become one whole that the latter is called the precious cauldron.

It is also said that about 1.3 inches under the navel is the cavity of real vitality (chen ch'i hsueh or lower tan t'ien) which lies between the front and back of the lower abdomen in proportion of seven to three and which is also called the golden stove (chin lu), the seat of (eternal) life.[2] Hence it is said that

[1] We hope this explanation will put an end to the usual dispute between Eastern and Western scholars, the former insisting that heart, and the latter that brain, is the seat of mind.
[2] The stove in the lower tan t'ien becomes the golden stove when it starts to transmute the generative force into vitality.

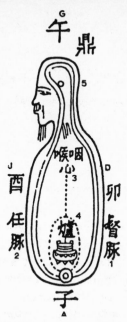

Figure 1 The four cardinal points: A bottom, G top, D back, J front
1 Channel of control (tu mo) 2 channel of function (jeu mo) 3
heart 4 stove 5 precious cauldron (See also figure 8, p. 141)

life is the generative force which develops in the genital organ.
The golden stove originally did not exist but comes into being
when the generative force develops and vitality manifests.

When the blood reaches the stove it changes into
negative generative force which originates from this centre.

Saliva flows from two channels under the tongue. If it
enters the jen mo channel (of function) it goes down into the
lower tan t'ien centre (under the navel) to change into negative
generative force, but a competent master should be sought to
teach the proper way of swallowing saliva;[3] otherwise it will

---

[3]Cf. *The Secrets of Chinese Meditation*, p. 206, first paragraph. Rider, London.

enter the stomach and intestines to be discharged as waste.

Question Will you please teach me the proper method of swallowing saliva?

Answer This is the quickest way to produce the generative force; it consists of touching the palate with the tongue to increase the flow of saliva more than usual. When the mouth is so full that you can hold no more and you are about to spurt it out, straighten your neck and swallow it. It will then enter the channel of function (jen mo) to reach the cavity of vitality (below the navel) where it will change into negative and positive generative force. When the generative force is full so will be the breath and when breath is full spirit is strong and your body will be robust.

If you have not been taught this proper method by a competent master, when you swallow saliva it will first enter the stomach and, after being digested, it will be driven into the heart and circulated in the blood vessels before reaching the channel of function where the blood gradually becomes grey white and sticky; it will produce the generative fluid which is harmful and disturbs the heart.

Since olden times many men and women have been ruined by the harmful effects of the generative fluid. When the genital duct dilates young women are liable to lose their virginity whereas men succumb easily to sexual desires and commit immoral acts.

When the penis stands during sleep at night this moment is called the hour tsu[4] and then it is most important to stop all

[4]According to the ancients the first half of the day is positive and the second half is negative. The first half begins at the hour tsu (between 11 p.m. and 1 a.m.) when the penis stands of itself during sleep in spite of the absence of thoughts and dreams. At the start of Tao practice, it is important to avail oneself of this moment when the penis stands to gather the generative force for sublimation, for the gathering of it during the negative half of the day is ineffective.

thoughts while gathering (ts'ai ch'u) the generative force (for sublimation). The gathering method differs with the age of each individual.

At puberty when (a youth has not indulged in sexual pleasures and his) body is still unimpaired, it will suffice to hold the vital force in the lower tan t'ien cavity (under the navel) and to concentrate on it for about ten months until its light manifests which is the moment for the macrocosmic alchemical agent's breakthrough to realise immortality. This is the quick method.

As to the middle-aged man, he should first repair the damage to his body caused by the dissipation of generative force. When the generative force and vitality are full again the light of vitality will manifest and his genital organ will become retractile which is the moment for the breakthrough. This is the slow method.

An old man over sixty-four whose positive principle has stopped developing, should practise the method of 'adding fuel' to prolong his life. If he knows it he should, when the penis erects, concentrate on checking it and start the breathing exercise to shrink it in a short while.

Question After the genital organ has not been aroused for a considerable time, what should one do if one does not practise the above method?

Answer This non-arousal shows that the generative force is exhausted; if it is not fully restored vitality will come to an end and death is not far off.

Question If the above method fails to check the arousal and erection of the penis, what should one do?

Answer If after practising it the penis does not shrink, quick and slow fires (i.e. the relevant breath rhythms) should be used with concentration on the cavity of mortality (sheng szu ch'iao) at the root of the penis until the penis is checked and brought under control. After it has shrunk the practiser should breathe *in* to drive the generative force into the base of the spine and thence up the backbone to the brain; and *out* to send it down to the lower tan t'ien centre (under the navel). Quick fire is produced by strong and slow fire by gentle breathing. It is most important that each complete breath should turn the generative force back to the source (below the navel) in order to put an end to the arousal of the penis.

My elder brother Kuei I Tsu said: 'When the positive vibrates and causes the penis to erect, one should breathe in and out to turn it back to the lower abdomen to nurture it.'

The patriarch Liu said: 'When the arousal occurs, practise the checking method and you will be satisfied with the result.'

Question The Tan Ching says: 'At eighty and even ninety if one meets a competent master one can still produce the golden elixir (of immortality).' If a man at sixty-four is devoid of the positive principle which has turned negative due to the gradual dissipation of his generative force over the preceding decades and can still restore his vitality so that he looks like a youth at sixteen, there must be some secret method which can restore the generative force. Will you please teach me?

Answer The patriarch Chang San Feng said: 'Old people who are impotent may use artificial means (e.g. masturbation) to arouse the genital organ. After its arousal one should gather the generative force from the vitality in the body. A man lives because of this vitality which produces the generative force, and dies when it is exhausted.'

Now study carefully the diagram on page 15 which is

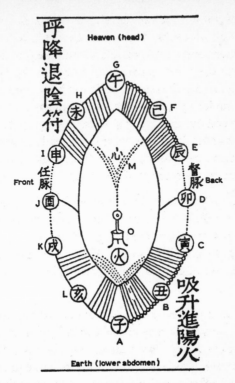

Figure 2 The microcosmic orbit and the channels of control and function A, G, D, J, are the four cardinal points of the microcosmic orbit A–B, A–C, A–E, A–F, are the four phases of ascent of positive fire in the channel of control G–H, G–I, G–K, G–A, are the four phases of descent of negative fire in the channel of function M Heart O Fire (in the stove)

very clear. As soon as the penis stands breathe in fresh air to fan the stove in the lower abdomen in order to drive the generative force into the channel of control (tu mo in the spine) and put it into microcosmic orbit.

Breathe in *nine times* to raise the generative force from position A to B.

If the penis continues to stand breathe in another *nine times* to raise the generative force from A to C. If the erection is not checked, then raise the generative force to D leaving it there for a little (for cleansing) before turning it back to the stove (in the lower abdomen).

Breathe in *nine times* again to raise the generative force from A to D leaving it there for a little before sending it up to E.

If the erection is still not checked breathe in a further *nine times* to raise the generative force from A to D leaving it there for a little before sending it up to F thence back to the stove.

You will thus complete four phases of nine breaths each or thirty-six in all, a positive number which controls the ascent of positive fire.

If in spite of these thirty-six breaths the genital organ is still aroused you should immediately gather the alchemical agent to collect vitality in order to restore the dissipated generative force.

To do this you should *breathe in* once more so that the generative force rises from A to D where it stops for a little before continuing up to G; no imagination is needed for this ascent. After the force has stopped at G for a little; *breathe out* imagining the generative force as descending from there to H, thence returning to the stove (via A) in *six descents*.

Then breathe *in* to let the generative force rise from A to G and *out* imagining it descend to I, thence returning to the stove in *six descents*.

Then breathe *in* to let the generative force rise from A to C and *out* imagining it descend to J where it stops for a little for purification before continuing to K thence returning to the stove in *six descents*.

Then breathe *in* once more to let the generative force rise from A to G and *out* to send it down to J and thence to A in *six descents*.

You will thus complete four phases of six descents each or twenty-four in all, a negative number which stands for the descent of negative fire.

The arousal of the genital organ feeds the inner fire in the stove which transforms the generative fluid derived from digestion of food into negative generative force to fortify the body and enliven spirit thereby lengthening the span of life.

Old and middle-aged people cannot practise alchemy without arousing the genital organ. When the penis stands, (essential) nature seated in the heart should be driven into the seat of (eternal) life below the navel to achieve their union by means of concentration.

Question What do you mean by the union of nature and life through concentration?

Answer This is uniting the negative breath in the heart with the positive breath in the lower abdomen. When the negative comes into contact with the positive breath, both heart and life will be set at rest in one place. When the positive breath in the lower abdomen meets the negative breath that comes down from the heart, the former will grow stronger.

Concentration consists of unifying the faculty of seeing in each eye to look into the lower tan t'ien cavity (under the navel) where (eternal) life will be held at a fixed spot. This is called the cultivation of both (essential) nature and (eternal) life (hsin ming shuang hsiu) to invigorate spirit and vitality. If your practice is successful you will in time experience congenial harmony in the lower abdomen, and all of a sudden the positive fire will soar up from the base of the spine to the top of the head when you breathe *in* and sink down to the centre of vitality in the lower tan t'ien (under the navel) when you breathe *out*. This is a full turn of the wheel of the law (or one microcosmic orbit).

You should now gather the aichemical agent for sublimation in conjunction with your concentration and in and out breathing; the penis will shrink and as you look into the cavity of vitality (the lower tan t'ien under the navel) you will in time see the light of vitality springing from this centre like a circle which proves that your body is full of generative and vital forces. This circle (of light) is the Supreme Ultimate (t'ai chi).

Your body came from your parents' thought of procreation but this circle existed before your body came into being since both your (essential) nature and (eternal) life were in it.

When you were a foetus in your mother's womb, your hands clasped your ears and your eyes were level with your bent knees. You did not breathe through your mouth and nose, and your breathing as well as your nature and life were subordinated to those of your mother. Although you did not eat you grew gradually. You were linked with your mother's womb by the umbilical cord. After about ten months in the womb, you were born into the world. Your body was soft like cotton but once the umbilical cord was cut, your prenatal foetal breathing stopped and was replaced by postnatal (usual) breath which then entered and left your body through your mouth and nostrils. From then on your faculty of seeing split into two and your tongue ceased to join up the channels of control and function (tu mo and jen mo). Your (essential) nature was carried by your postnatal breath up to the heart which became its seat, and your (eternal) life down to the lower abdomen to stay there. The space between (essential) nature and (eternal) life was a little over eight inches. Since spirit was displaced by consciousness the latter has controlled you from childhood to adulthood and old age, and alas your nature and life will never unite again.

Since vitality increases in weight by sixty-four chu[5] every thirty-two months, when a baby is two years and eight months old, he has developed a unit of positive principle (yang) with his vitality weighing sixty-four chu. When he is five years and four months old, the positive principle increases to two units while vitality gains another sixty-four chu. At eight, the positive principle increases to three units with vitality gaining another sixty-four chu. When he is ten years and eight months old, the positive principle increases to four units while vitality gains another sixty-four chu. When he is thirteen years and four months old, the positive principle has five units while vitality increases by another sixty-four chu. At sixteen, the positive principle contains six units while vitality increases by another sixty-four chu. (Thus the total weight of vitality is 384 chu).

If the twenty-four chu inherited from his parents are added to the 360 chu derived from heaven and earth, the total is also 384 chu, or one catty, and he whose vitality weighs 384 chu lives.

But at the age of sixteen his consciousness takes over the control of his life, and his intellect develops gradually. With inner fire soaring up in his body, his (essential) nature is replaced by his heart so that desires and passions fill his being. And in his quest for fame and wealth he indulges in cunning and artfulness and invents all sorts of tricks to deceive others without appreciating that by so doing he harms his real nature. So by troubling his heart and body, he dissipates his vitality and causes his (essential) nature to vacillate.

As a result his span of life shortens, and with his gate of mortality wide open and real nature impaired, his vital force

---

[5]Chu = a weight equal to the twenty-fourth part of a tael, which is the Chinese ounce, equal to 1⅓ oz. avoirdupois.

flows out like running water. So gambling away his (essential) nature with wine and sex, he allows his generative and vital forces to drain away and he is dragged into mortality.

Thus his positive (yang) vitality decreases gradually while the negative counterpart (yin) grows in proportion so that he becomes a mortal worldling.

From his sixteenth year onward a unit of negative principle develops every ninety-six months. So at twenty-four another unit of negative principle develops and through not nurturing vitality he loses sixty-four chu of it. At thirty-two the negative principle increases to two units and through not preventing the waste of vitality he loses another sixty-four chu of it. At forty the negative principle increases to three units since he does not repent his foolishness, he loses another sixty-four chu of vitality. At forty-eight the negative principle increases to four units and through not making up for the loss of vitality, the latter is gradually exhausted in his lower abdomen causing his hair and beard to turn grey; he again loses another sixty-four chu of it. At fifty-six the negative principle increases to five units; and since he continues giving way to worldly pleasures and looking for fame and wealth, his liver gradually weakens, his sight becomes bad, his memory fails and his constitution withers; if in spite of this he still refuses to wake up he again loses another sixty-four chu of vitality. At sixty-four the negative principle increases to six units; if he still does not realise his mortality, he continues dreaming until his hair is white, his energy exhausted and his features emaciated, and he again loses another sixty-four chu. Being now unable to reproduce the generative force to sustain his body, all his 384 chu of vitality are exhausted with death fast closing in.

Chapter 1 teaches the method of fixing spirit in its original cavity (tsu ch'iao in the centre of the brain between and behind the eyes) so that when the generative force vibrates in the condition of utter stillness, it can be gathered to fortify the body and prolong life.

If the generative force is gathered for a hundred (successive) days, sixty-four chu of vitality is gained and a unit of positive principle is produced; this is like 'adding fuel' to feed and prolong life.

With the same determination, if the generative force is gathered for another hundred days an additional sixty-four chu of vitality are gained while the positive principle is increased to two units; the body now becomes very strong and all ailments vanish.

If the gathering of generative force continues for another hundred days an additional sixty-four chu of vitality are gained with the positive increased to three units; all cavities in the body are cleared for rejuvenation, and the practiser's steps are light and quick with clear sight and good hearing.

With continuous advance for another hundred days, another sixty-four chu of vitality are gained with the positive principle increased to four units; the practiser now feels very comfortable like a wealthy man who has all the means to enjoy life; his skin is lustrous and his white hair turns black (as before).

After another hundred days, a further sixty-four chu of vitality are gained while the positive principle increases to five units; his spirits are very high and new teeth grow to replace the fallen ones.

After yet another hundred days, another sixty-four chu of vitality are gained with the positive principle increased to six units; he enjoys the cream of life while restoring (his body) fully to its all-positive state in early infancy and regaining the circle of t'ai chi (or Supreme Ultimate) wherein real positive vitality and essential nature unite to emit the light of vitality which is the light of true nature in the precious cauldron (in the head) and that of true life in the stove (in the lower abdomen). Students should ponder over all this carefully.

Question You have said that the method of producing true generative force differs according to the three categories of practisers: the chaste youth, the middle-aged and the old man; will you please teach me how to distinguish the genuine from spurious generative force?

Answer The first step is to fix spirit in its original cavity (tsu ch'iao in the centre of the brain between and behind the eyes) by concentration so that the light of vitality manifests in the ensuing condition of utter stillness. In this absence of thoughts, the positive principle will in time manifest causing the penis to erect. The practiser should now wipe out the concept of the self so as to free his heart from disturbances, and then concentrate on his spirit to drive it into the centre of vitality (the lower tan t'ien below the navel); this is the immersion of fire in water. The element of water in the lower belly is thus scorched by spirit's fire and thereby transmuted into true vitality. The practiser should gather immediately the true generative force.

If he does not know how to take advantage of the absence of thoughts in this condition of stillness to gather true vitality when the positive manifests (causing the penis to stand up) he will give rise to sexual desire which will transform the generative force into postnatal generative fluid which (is useless and) cannot be gathered. In this event he should breathe in and out quickly through the nostrils to turn back the positive principle (so that it will not scatter). This breathing is not to gather the (flowing) generative fluid (caused by his misuse) of the manifestations of the positive principle.

Students should pay careful attention to all this.

If the practiser sets his mind intentionally on gathering the generative force (i.e. if he is mindful of it and so fails to empty his mind of all thoughts) he will never produce the golden elixir.

3

CLEARING THE EIGHT PSYCHIC CHANNELS[1]

When beginners first sit in meditation they always complain that because they cannot move their loins and legs they develop cramp and their nerves are on edge, the circulation of the blood and (vital) breath is blocked and the ensuing pains and numbness become unbearable.

[1]The eight main psychic channels: (1) the tu mo or channel of control rises from the base of the penis and passes through the coccyx up the backbone to the brain; (2) the jen mo or channel of function rises from the base of the penis and goes up along the belly, passes through the navel, the pit of the stomach, the chest and throat, before going up to the brain; (3) the tai mo or belt channel from both sides of the navel forms a belt which circles the belly; (4) the ch'ung mo or thrusting channel rises from the base of the penis, goes up between the tu mo and jen mo channels and ends in the heart; (5) the yang yu or positive arm channels in the outer sides of both arms link both shoulders with the centres of the palms after passing through the middle fingers; (6) the yin yu or negative arm channels in the inner sides of both arms link the centres of the palms with the chest; (7) the yang chiao or positive leg channels rise from the centres of the soles and turn along the outer sides of the ankles and legs before reaching the base of the penis where they connect other channels; and (8) the yin chiao or negative leg channels rise from the centres of the soles and turn along the inner sides of the ankles and legs before reaching the base of the penis where they connect other channels. These eight main channels, when free from obstructions, are interlocked to form with their ramifications, a network through which the generative force flows freely and then the vital breath circulates unrestrictedly.

This chapter deals with the method of restoring free circulation of the blood to put an abrupt end to numbness in the limbs.

The eight (main) psychic channels (when free from obstructions, together with their ramifications are interlocked to form a network which) play two distinct roles: (a) the unimpeded flow of generative force and (b) the unrestricted circulation of vital breath.

(a) *The unimpeded flow of generative force*

The free flow of generative force through (the network formed by) the eight psychic channels (and their ramifications) is dealt with first.

The base of these eight psychic channels is the cavity or gate of mortality (sheng szu ch'iao at the root of the penis) which is linked with the the base of the spine by the channel of control (tu mo) which then rises in the backbone up to the occiput before entering the ni wan or brain.

From the centre of the brain the channel of function (jen mo which has joined the tu mo in the brain) descends in the medulla oblongata to link with the hsuan ying cavity (the mysterious bridle behind the heavenly pool in the palate) which is connected by a fork with the upper jawbone where true vitality (see note 4 page 7) can (easily) find an outlet to disperse. Under the hsuan ying cavity is the throat by which the channel of function goes down in the pulmonary artery, the right ventricle of the heart, the hepatic artery under the diaphragm where is a cavity called chiang kung (or the solar plexus) which is under the heart, thence down to the cavity of vitality (or the lower tan t'ien below the navel) before reaching the testicles from which it returns to the cavity of mortality (at the root of the penis).

These two (vertical) channels (tu mo and jen mo) cut across the belt channel (tai mo) linking it with the heart above, the generative or genital gate (yang kuan, the opening at the end of the penis by which the generative fluid and urine flow out) below, the navel in front, the kidneys behind and the thrusting channel (ch'ung mo) in the middle of the body.

This (roughly) describes how the (four) psychic channels are interlinked for the production, circulation, discharge and purification of the generative force.

When these channels are blocked, the generative force cannot be produced and the man gradually grows old, like a lamp which ceases to give light for lack of oil because without the generative force the human body perishes. Therefore, the practiser should call on enlightened masters for instruction on how to generate and transmute the generative force, get rid of ailments and prolong life.

Question You have spoken of the production, flow, emission and purification of the generative force; will you please explain all this in detail?

Answer The method of producing the generative force is for people over sixty-four whose body is wholly negative. They should read Chapter 2 and practise the method to produce the generative force in order to strengthen the (vital) breath.

To transmute the generative force consists of raising it (in the tu mo) from the base of and up the spine to the back of the head and the ni wan or brain, thence lowering it in (the jen mo) to the hsuan ying cavity (behind the heavenly pool in the palate), the throat, the chiang kung cavity (the solar plexus) and then to the lower tan t'ien (under the navel); this is the microcosmic orbiting (or turning the wheel of the law) a few of which will suffice for the purpose.

In case of nocturnal emission one should practise the method taught in Chapter 10 in order to stop it entirely.

The method of purifying the generative force is taught in Chapter 6 and consists of sending the positive fire (yang huo) up and the negative fire (yin fu) down in order to transmute the generative force into prenatal vitality. You should pay careful attention to the above four methods so that you can combine them for profitable use; and if you succeed, you will understand more than half of the science of alchemy.

(b) *The unrestricted circulation of vital breath*

Question Will you please teach me how to get rid of numbness in the legs which annoys me when I sit in meditation?

Answer The (vital) breath circulates in the (network of) eight (main) psychic channels whose base is the mortal gate (sheng szu ch'iao at the root of the penis) which is linked to the brain above and the soles of the feet below. The breath either accumulates or disperses solely because of this cavity. If the blood circulates freely in the body and (vital) breath is strong, the positive principle (yang) grows causing the negative (yin) to decline; the element of fire will develop in that of water and 'flowers will blossom in the snow'. The whole body will be rejuvenated through this cavity of mortality which is the centre that produces vitality and which ordinary men ignore in spite of its daily functioning. If its duct is weakened a man's weak voice will immediately betray its lack of support by vitality and become like that of a woman. His heart will waver and he will act indecisively; he will be like a eunuch.

The cavity of mortality is the source of a man's vigour: it is not only a place where the alchemical agent (the generative force) is gathered but also the seat of courage which is instrumental to correct thinking, radiant mien, rejuvenation and robustness. When the blood and (vital) breath circulate freely in the body all ailments vanish.

This cavity of mortality (at the root of the penis) is the source from which (vital) breath circulates in all parts of the body. Therefore, each morning, after leaving your bed you should circulate this (vital) breath in all the eight psychic channels. This consists of stopping breathing through the nose and mouth in order to concentrate on the cavity of mortality as the point of departure (in the following ten phases of breathing):

1 Breathe in to drive the (vital) breath into the channel of control (tu mo in the spinal column) from its base up to the brain.

2 Breathe out to lower the (vital) breath in the channel of function (jen mo in front of the body) and return it to the mortal cavity (at the base of the penis).

3 Breathe in to raise it (in the jen mo or channel of function) from the mortal cavity to the cavity of vitality (or lower tan t'ien) and to the navel where the tai mo or belt channel starts from both sides of the navel forming a belt (which circles the belly) and where the (vital) breath divides into two to reach the small of the back, thence going up to both shoulders where it stops.

4 Breathe out to let it flow from both shoulders down into the (positive) yang yu channels in the outer sides of both wrists to the middle fingers before reaching the centres of both palms where it stops.

5 Breathe in to lift the (vital) breath from the centres of both palms into the (negative) yin yu channels in the inner sides of both wrists up to the chest where it stops.

6 Breathe out to drive the (vital) breath down to the belt channel where its two branches re-unite before returning to the mortal cavity.

7 Breathe in to lift it from the mortal cavity into the thrusting channel (ch'ung mo) up to the chiang kung cavity (solar plexus under the heart) where it stops; on no account should it rise above the heart.

8 Breathe out to send it from under the heart down to the mortal cavity where it divides into two to descend in the two positive ch'iao channels on the outer sides of the thighs and through the toes of the feet before reaching the centres of the soles of the feet, called bubbling spring cavities (yung ch'uan) where it stops.

9 Breathe in to raise it from the soles of the feet into the negative ch'iao channels in the inner sides of the legs up to the mortal cavity and thence to the cavity of vitality (below the navel) where it stops.

10 Breathe out to lower it from the cavity of vitality to the mortal cavity where it stops.

The (vital) breath should circulate in all the eight psychic channels in order to clear all cavities of negative impurities which hinder the preparation of the golden elixir.

If the above exercise is done daily causing (vitality to) vibrate in the channels, this shows that they are cleared of all impurities. If they are not cleared, the negative impurities cannot be eliminated and the alchemical agent cannot be gathered. Even if this agent were gathered, it would not produce the elixir of life. You should pay particular attention to all this.

Question You have spoken of the free circulation of (vital) breath in all eight psychic channels, but each time I wanted to sit longer my numb legs prevented me. Will you please teach me how to stop this numbness?

Answer When you sit in meditation and feel the legs numb, this is because you are not accustomed to the posture. The numbness becomes unbearable because this posture exerts pressure on and blocks the blood vessels and psychic channels thereby obstructing the free circulation of blood and (vital) breath. If you want relief you should shut your mouth and stop breathing, raise the feet and knock the ground with the heels; then breathe in to lift the (vital) breath from the centres of the soles of the feet through the yin ch'iao channels (on the inner sides of the thighs) up to the lower tan t'ien centre (beneath the navel) and breathe out to drive it down through the yang ch'iao channels (on the outside of the legs) to the centres of the soles. Repeat this exercise a few times and the numbness will disappear.

4

GATHERING THE MICROCOSMIC OUTER ALCHEMICAL AGENT[1]

The human body is like a rootless tree and relies solely on the breath as root and branches. A lifetime is just a dream, like an out breath which does not guarantee the in breath after it, and today does not insure the morrow. If life is passed aimlessly with death ever coming unexpectedly, the bones of the body will disperse, the four elements (of metal, wood, water and fire) will scatter (see note 3 on page 36) and the deluded consciousness (or thought, see *figure 4* on page 35) will transmigrate through another realm of existence without knowing what form it will take in another life. So birth and death will alternate in endless aeons in which the subject will remain ignorant and will delight in laziness without a chance to awaken to Reality.

Now that you have heard about the precious teaching do not go away empty-handed. (If you do not listen to it) you will not escape from illness and death when you grow old and will thus waste a lifetime in the human world.

Therefore, take a bold resolution and start to train seriously. As from today you should dwell in singleness of

[1]The outer alchemical agent is produced by means of fresh air breathed in and out to transmute the generative force into vitality.

thought; your eyes and ears should disengage from their objects; regulate your diet; reduce your sleep; refrain from futile talk and jokes; stop thinking and worrying; cast away soft comfort and cease to discriminate between the handsome and the ugly so that you can be like the cicada feeding on dew to preserve its unsullied body and like the tortoise absorbing vitality from sunlight to enjoy long life.

You should gather (vital) breath in the morning and sublimate it in the evening; if you do not so practise you will miss your good luck.

Therefore, alchemy consists first in controlling the heart (the seat of fire) so that it cannot be stirred by the seven emotions (pleasure, anger, sorrow, joy, love, hate and desire) and upset by the five thieves; the six sense organs are immobilised and the generative force cannot be easily aroused.

The five thieves are: the eye, ear, nose, tongue and body. When the eyes see a form the love of it steals the generative force; when the ears hear a sound the desire for it stirs the generative force; when the nose smells fragrance covetousness of it dissipates the generative force; when the tongue tastes food fondness for it drains the generative force away; and when the body feels touch, stupidity arises to injure the generative force. If these five thieves are allowed to injure the body day and night, what will remain of the generative force? If it flows away spirit is bound to disperse and the body will perish.

A practiser should regard his body as a country and the generative force as its population. Unstirred generative force ensures security for the population, and the fullness of spirit and (vital) breath increases the prosperity of the country. Likewise in his quest for immortality he should fight hard with the enemy to achieve prenatal vitality.

Question What is the meaning of the terms 'laying the foundation' (chu chi) and self-purification (lien chi)?

Answer Before 'laying the foundation', spirit wanders outside in quest of sense data, vitality dissipates and the generative force is corrupt. You should sublimate the three precious elements, namely the generative force, (vital) breath and spirit to restore their original strength, and the foundation will be laid when these three elements unite; only then can immortality be attained.

This foundation will lift you from the worldly to the saintly plane, still your spirit within ten months, and enable you to give up sleep within nine or ten months, dispense with food and drink within ten months, feel neither cold in winter nor hot in summer, and achieve unperturbed spirit which leads to stable serenity.

If (vital) breath is purified it will settle and need neither inhalation nor exhalation for hundreds and thousands of aeons. If spirit is purified it will be immaterial, free from either dullness that causes sleepiness or stirring that leads to wandering.

This laying of the foundation will cause life to last as long as heaven and earth and lead to the acquisition of the supernatural powers possessed by all the immortals. By laying the foundation of positive spirit is meant stopping the positive generative force from draining away, and thus producing the golden elixir. All this is achieved by laying the foundation.

The body, heart and thought are called 'three families' (san chia) and the generative force, (vital) breath and spirit are called the three treasures (san pao) or three basic elements (san yuan). Body, heart and thought stand for the principal (chu), and the generative force, (vital) breath and spirit for

The inferior realm of desire: The generative force sublimated into vitality – the positive extracted from the negative.

The medium realm of form: Vitality sublimated into spirit – developing the positive to eliminate the negative gradually.

The superior realm beyond form: Full development of the positive to eradicate the negative completely – spirit returned to nothingness.

Figure 3 The three realms of desire, form and beyond form.

function (yung). The union of the three elements into one whole produces the elixir of immortality.

The three elements (or factors) can be controlled and returned to the one source only in the condition of serene voidness. When the heart is empty of externals spirit and nature unite; and when the body is still, the generative force and passions are extinct. When thought is reduced to the state of serenity, the three factors mingle into one.

When passion and nature unite this is called the union of the elements of metal (chin) and wood (mu). When the generative force and spirit unite this is called the mingling of the elements of water and fire. When thought is stabilised, this is the fullness of the five elements (metal, wood, water, fire and earth).

The generative force changes into vitality when the body is motionless; vitality changes into spirit when the heart is

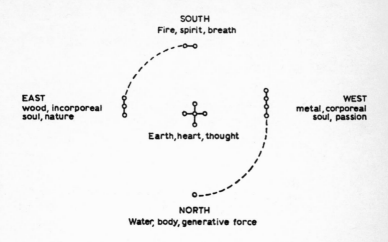

Figure 4 The perfect union (See also figure 8, p. 141).71

unstirred; and spirit returns to nothingness because of immutable thought.

If the heart does not move, three (vital) breaths of the east and two of the south unite to total five forms. (See fig. 4 for explanation.) If the body does not move, one (vital) breath of the north and four of the west unite to total five. If thought does not move the centre begets all five (vital) breaths. When body, heart and thought are all motionless the three families meet to beget the immortal foetus.

One vitality first divides in two, the positive and negative which, by taking fixed positions, then beget the five elements, each in a different location. Hence the element of earth causes that of metal to develop, that of wood to prosper, that of water to stop and that of fire to cease.

Only the saints and sages know the method of reversing the mechanism of life to return to its very source. To restore the one source they gather up the five,[2] harmonise the four,[3] a assemble the three,[4] and unite the two[5] divisions of one vitality.

For if the body does not move, the generative force is strong enough to turn the element of water back to its source. If the heart is unstirred (vital) breath is strong enough to turn back the element of fire. If (essential) nature is still, the incorporeal (soul) lies hidden to let the element of wood return to its source. If passion subsides the corporeal (soul) is overcome and the element of metal returns. If the four elements (of metal, wood, water and fire)[6] are in harmony thought is held to the element of earth which then returns to its source. This is the return of all five (vital) breaths to their source in the brain (or ni wan), which is the union of the three treasures (note 4 below) into one whole for self-purification.

Question I have read the Hui Ming Ching and Chin Hsien Ching Lun about blocking the genital duct to purify the outflowing alchemical agent until the practiser is aware of its production. The patriarch Li Hsu An also said: 'When busy snatch a rest to gather the outer agent.' Han Chung Li said: 'This is blocking the genital gate (yang kuan or the opening at the end of the penis).' Ch'ung Hsu Tsu said: 'Sublimate (the agent) until you are

[2] The five elements of metal, wood, water, fire and earth. See also note 3.
[3] The four components are: body, breath, incorporeal and corporeal souls symbolised respectively by the elements of water, fire, wood and metal of the four cardinal points of the microcosmic orbit: south, north, east and west. When the four unite with the element of earth at the centre which stands for thought (concentration) this is called the harmony of the four components.
The Hsin Ming Kuei Chih says: 'When the eyes cease seeing the incorporeal soul is in the liver; when the ears cease hearing the generative force is in the lower abdomen; when the tongue ceases moving, spirit is in the heart and when the nose ceases smelling the corporeal soul is in the lungs. When the four organs are perfect, the four components unite with earth at the centre.'
[4] The generative force, vitality and spirit.
[5] The positive yang and negative yin.
[6] See note 3.

perfectly aware of it and then you will produce true vitality.' I do not know the blocking method; please teach me.

Answer Lao Tsu said: 'Baseness is the root of nobility and inferiority is the foundation of superiority.' Postnatal nourishing and restoring pertain to the base and inferior method. That which is base is referred to by the master as something that can cause one to blush with shame and that which is inferior is something on the ground to be picked up.

The Hsin Ming Kuei Chih says: 'Past immortals refused to reveal it because to disclose it is extremely laughable.' The Tan Ching says: 'To speak of the root of nature and life and of the mortal cavity is to make the speaker blush with shame, and although the method is profound, it can cause Homeric laughter.'

Now to block the genital duct gathers the (outer) flowing agent and is like carving an inscription on a stone tablet; the stone mason uses tools to carve it until the characters are formed and then carefully polishes it. If the generative force is not purified prenatal vitality will not develop; if so when can you gather the microcosmic outer (alchemical) agent to make good the loss of generative fluid?

You should ponder over all this and when the microcosmic outer (alchemical) agent is gathered spirit is (i.e. you are) aware of it. When the generative and vital forces burst out causing your body to shiver a little, you should press your middle finger on the mortal cavity (at the base of the penis) to ascertain the quantity of generative force that flows out and the amount retained: that is when it divides in two parts, one draining off in liquid form that can produce offspring while the other is returned to the channel of control (tu mo in the spine) wherein it will be purified to become vitality which can later be transmuted into the elixir of immortality.

The Chin Hsien Ching Lun's second chapter says: 'The generative force is the most precious thing for the human body that contains it lives and the body without it dies; because it nourishes and preserves the root of (essential) nature and (eternal) life. No worldly men know how to produce and purify it. If it is exhausted it should be restored by the reproducing process; this is called restoring the generative force to invigorate the brain.'

My book, though written colloquially, is for the benefit of practisers who should read this chapter carefully; those of high spirituality who strive to advance progressively will achieve immortality whereas those of little determination can at least prolong their span of life and so enjoy longevity, for this chapter is also a precious guide to improve health.

Now let us discuss again the process of gathering and purifying the (microcosmic outer) alchemical agent. Can this agent be really produced and what is the proper time to gather it?

You should not only know when this agent is not being made but also distinguish its premature from its overdue production. For the mere gathering of deficient vitality leads to no result; you will not avoid death and your long efforts will be in vain. Therefore, it is most important to produce and sublimate the (microcosmic outer) alchemical agent.

The immortal Ts'ao Huan Yang said: 'Even when you are busy relax a little to sublimate the outer agent in order to gather prenatal vitality from nothingness.'

Lu Tsu said: 'Do not relax efforts until the (microcosmic outer) aichemical agent is produced and spirit is aware of its presence.' By 'spirit being aware of the alchemical agent' is meant knowing whether the process of production is efficient or not. If vitality is felt to be deficient you should not hastily gather this agent but should wait until vitality is fully developed; only then can the generative force be transmuted into vitality to invigorate the brain.

Vitality is basically adequate in the human body but dissipates because of sexual indulgence; hence its deficiency. To make good such dispersion it is necessary to use the (microcosmic outer) alchemical agent to reproduce vitality in sufficient quantity for use. If the agent is not pure, genuine and complete, how can it be employed to restore vitality? If the heart is affected by sexual desire the generative force becomes sullied and changes into postnatal generative fluid which cannot be used as a (microcosmic outer) alchemical agent. If (vital) breath is incomplete the agent is young (and weak) and cannot be transmuted into the elixir of life. Hence the necessity of sublimating the (microcosmic outer) alchemical agent.

The genital organ is also aroused and stands erect in the absence of sexual desire; this is due to the postnatal generative force vibrating in the body (to seek an outlet) and also to the inadequate circulation of fire during your meditation which fails to reach and check the penis.

Hence the method of correct breathing to circulate quick fire up and down (in the microcosmic orbit) and so immobilise the generative force causing the genital organ to retract (thus stopping the drain of vitality). This secret of sublimation consists in one word 'knowledge', that is knowledge of the process which depends on the age of the practiser and the amount of vitality dissipated, and should not work at random. For this loss of vitality may be little or large; the prenatal vitality may be deficient or adequate; and both postnatal and prenatal generative forces may have or may not have dispersed; hence the process of sublimation is not the same for all practisers.

Question You have mentioned numbers such as thirty-six for each or 216 for all six phases of the ascent of positive fire, and twenty-four for each or 144 for all six phases of the descent of negative fire, this is 360 for each complete microcosmic orbiting; and you have also said they are symbolic only and do not mean counting the breath 360 times. On which basis should sublimation be made?

Answer The number 360 stands for an inhalation and an exhalation that makes a complete breath. The rise (of the generative and vital forces) in the back bone is called the ascent of positive fire and the fall down the front of the body is called the descent of negative fire.

When breathing in, the heart, spirit and thought should rise together from the base of the spine at the cardinal point A (at the root of the penis. *See figure* 2 on page 15) to the intermediate points B and C before reaching D where they are held up for a short pause for cleansing, and thence to the cardinal point G (the top of the head); this involves six phases of rise (A, B, C, D, E, F) in the channel of control (tu mo in the spine) and is called the ascent of positive fire.

When breathing out, the heart, spirit and thought should together go down from the brain at the cardinal point G to the intermediate points H and I before reaching J where they pause a little for purification, and thence to A; this involves six negative phases of descent in the channel of function (jen mo) to return vitality to the source and is called the descent of negative fire.

So these positive ascents and negative descents are caused by in and out breathing.

When the generative and vital forces start vibrating (in the lower tan t'ien cavity under the navel) you should breathe in – this is to close (ho) the respiratory mechanism (so that the air goes down to exert pressure on the lower abdomen); and at the same time by rolling your eyes up you should follow the ascent of generative force and vitality from the bottom to the top of the head, thus:

G ↖

Eyes   D

A ↗

When you breathe out, you should open (p'i) the respiratory mechanism so that the air goes out of the body (to relax pressure on the lower abdomen); at the same time your eyes should follow the descent of generative force and vitality from the top to the bottom, thus:

↙ G

J ↙   Eyes

↘ A

So to complete an orbit you should roll your eyes right round thus:

↙ G ↖

J   Eyes   D

↘ A ↗

All this is generally called the ascent of positive and descent of negative fire; while inhalation, shutting, ascent and opening, exhalation, descent are the phases of the alchemical process.

As for the bellows (t'o yo, see page 43), it is used to make these ascents and descents. Prenatal vitality is produced and stored up by this (breathing) process while (fire in) the heart and (water in the) lower abdomen mingle. If the generative and vital forces do not vibrate (in the lower abdomen) there is no need to employ the inner bellows. For ventilation (by in and out breathing), the ascent of positive and descent of negative fire, the cauldron and stove, are so-called and come into play only after the generative and vital forces have vibrated.

The six phases of each microcosmic orbiting have their fixed positions without which the elixir of immortality cannot be prepared. They start rising from the mortal cavity A (at the root of the penis) to D and G *(see figure 2,* on page 15) which are the first, second and third positions in the ascent; and then go down from G (at the top of the head) to J and A which are the first, second and third positions in the descent. These are the six phases of the microcosmic orbit.

The process of gathering the (microcosmic outer) alchemical agent is thus: when the generative and vital forces vibrate press your middle finger on the cavity of mortality, and as soon as their mechanism starts moving, breathe in and out to raise a gentle breeze (sun feng or ventilation) which causes the prenatal generative and vital forces to go up in the tu mo (in the spine) and down in the jen mo (in the head and the front side of the chest and body) to make a full rotation.

Your eyes, head and limbs should be waiting for this unusual experience which is the most difficult thing for a beginner. However, after it has happened a few times, you will be automatically ready to take the correct attitude without even knowing why and what makes you do so.

As the wheel of the law (fa lun, i.e. the microcosmic orbit) turns round, it causes the generative and vital forces to go down (in the jen mo channel) to return to the lower tan t'ien (under the navel). All this takes place automatically; then where is the difficulty?

But never try to gather fresh air to make good the dissipation of generative force and so restore vitality in the body, which is sheer nonsense. You should call on an enlightened master and ask him to teach you about the gentle breeze (sun feng), bellows (t'o yo), shutting and opening (ho p'i), the six phases (liu hou), the ascent of the positive (chin yang) and descent of the negative principle (tui yin) and the cleansing and purifyinging (mu yu).

Question You have said that the gentle breeze, using the bellows, shutting and opening, the six phases of the ascent of positive and descent of negative fire, cleansing and purifying all pertain to microcosmic purification. I am clear about this but am afraid that future students will have difficulty in understanding the teaching. I hope you will explain it in a book for the benefit of posterity so that spurious teachers and imposters cannot deceive and mislead the coming generations.

Answer The gentle breeze (sun feng) is postnatal in and out breathing through the nostrils. Each intake of fresh air pushes up the positive vitality (in the channel of control in the spine or tu mo); this is called ascent. The following exhalation releases the pressure so that vitality goes down (in the channel of function in the front of the body or jen mo); this is called descent. Each ascent is from the base of the spine to the ni wan or brain and each descent is from the brain to the cavity of mortality (shen szu ch'iao at the root of the penis). All this is caused by the gentle breeze.

The bellows (t'o yo) or the bagpipe works in the body; it cannot be found in the absence of the generative and vital forces and manifests only when vitality vibrates under the navel. The bag is above and the pipe is below; the space between them is about 8·4 inches, the bag being where (essential) nature is seated (in the heart) and the pipe where life is (under the navel).

When postnatal (fresh) air is breathed in prenatal vital force goes up (in the channel of control); this is the shutting (ho) process which consists of breathing in outside air, thus closing the respiratory mechanism so that the air goes down in the body to push up prenatal vital force thus clearing all psychic channels. It causes life which is below to unite with (essential) nature which is above.

When postnatal fresh air is breathed out prenatal vital force (now released from pressure) goes down (in the channel of function); this is the opening (p'i) process which consists of expelling air by the nostrils to let prenatal vital force return to its source (under the navel), thus clearing all psychic channels. It causes (essential) nature which is above to unite with life which is below.

During this process of sublimation you should roll your (closed) eyes to look successively at the four cardinal points A, D, G, J (and A) thus:

$$\begin{array}{ccc} \nwarrow & 1G3 & \nearrow \\ 2J \searrow & \text{Eyes} & \nearrow D2 \\ & 3A1 & \end{array}$$

This is called inner and outer ho p'i (i.e. inner vital force and outer air) which operate like a bellows. Although the mechanism is the same the air in the body works differently from that in the bellows. While the inner breeze starts the eyes roll to look at the four cardinal points A, D, G and J, and while nature and life in the body change place during the shutting and opening process, the latter sets in motion the generative force which is automatically transmuted into vitality (which circulates up and down). Even the practiser himself does not know why the head, eyes, limbs and breathing function like this, for each inhalation followed by the shutting, and each exhalation preceded by the opening, takes place spontaneously.

The natural six phases of orbiting are: ascent from A, cleansing at D, stay at G, descent from G, purification at J and return to A; they are caused by an inhalation which initiates the ascent and an exhalation the descent.

Thus the rise from A to D and G involves the first, second and third stages of an ascent, and the fall from G to J and A comprises the first, second and third stages of a descent. Hence the Tan Ching says: 'Execute three phases up the back and another three down the front of the body, pick up and return (the vital force) to the lower tan t'ien cavity (under the navel).'

The six phases in the ascent of positive fire from A to B, C, D, E and F are positive; the positive number being nine, the total number of all six positive phases is: 9 x 4 (for the four changing seasons) x 6 (phases) = 216.

The six phases in the descent of its negative counterpart from G to H, I, J, K and L are negative: the negative number being six, the total number of all six negative phases is: 6 x 4 x 6 = 144.

Since the two cardinal points D and J are reserved for cleansing and purification and are, therefore, not taken into consideration, actually the total positive number is 180 and the total negative number is 120. So both ascent and descent involve 300 breaths which are symbolic only (and not actual counts).

My master Liao K'ung said: 'Practise this every morning and evening in order to avoid all risks (wei hsien) at night (e.g. involuntary emission).'

Question Every day I turn the water-wheels (ho che) (i.e. the microcosmic orbits) but still cannot stop involuntary emission; what is the reason?

Answer According to your statement this is purposeless turning of empty water-wheels which is unprofitable. You asked before about the gentle breeze, using the bellows, shutting and opening, the six phases of ascent and descent, cleansing and purification; these stages are involved in each in and out breath. The method should begin when the penis erects at night and consists of blocking the genital gate with pointed concentration in order to drive spirit into the cavity of vitality (under the navel). This is like a blacksmith using his bellows; the air from it blows the inner fire which, becoming intense, transmutes the generative force into vitality. The latter is then gathered and sent up and down in the microcosmic orbit.

At present you just sit motionless, close your eyes and then make the ascents and descents 360 times; this is purposeless turning of empty water-wheels and is not the proper method of preparing the golden elixir. It is because when you began to meditate your mind was disturbed by thoughts that you were taught to make 360 turns to achieve mental stillness only. Your body is now so weak that if you fail to restore the generative force you will not be able to improve your health.

5

QUICK AND SLOW FIRES

Quick and slow fires are postnatal heat used to cure illnesses and prolong life and also to unite the sun with the moon (i.e. the positive yang and negative yin).[1]

The method consists of using postnatal fire to draw out prenatal fire[2] so that both unite in order to extract from food and drink the sweet dew (kan lu or pure saliva) which descending in the channel of function (jen mo in the front of the body) changes into negative generative force and helps to produce the latter.

Slow fire is produced by (a meditative method which consists of) closing both eyes to develop a mind which, although void, does not cease to work: which, although radiant, does not continue (to abide); and which is neither forgotten nor upheld. The time set for using quick and slow fires should be in the proportion of three to seven.

---

[1]The sun stands for the positive and the moon for the negative principle.
[2]Prenatal and postnatal fires are respectively spiritual or positive fire that existed before birth and its corrupt counterpart or negative fire after birth.

My master teaching me the use of quick and slow fires said: 'Quick fire shifts and slow fire calms.' Both fires are used to transform impurities in the viscera into tears which are discharged; to achieve the harmony of the four components[3], the union of the five elements[4] and their return to the root; and to turn back the inner light to shine upon itself which unites the sun with the moon.[5]

No known immortals on earth suffer from tuberculosis or take medicine to cure ailments or improve their health. Now that you are determined to seek immortality you should quickly eradicate all the ailments latent in the body; and it will not be late to practise the Tao after you are free of all of them. The saints and sages of old did not wait for illnesses to manifest and then cured them; they cured them while they were latent.

If you look at people they all seem to be in good health and free from sickness but in reality they have in their bodies the roots of illness which have not yet developed. It is regrettable that they only look for pleasures without realising their mistakes and errors. They always give rise to stupidity by seeking comfortable houses, drinking strong wines, enjoying exciting music and dances and giving themselves up to pleasures. They do not realise that attractive forms can disturb their seeing, that music and songs can mislead their hearing and that going to bed when they are drunk and full of food can cause their generative force to disperse. Their health declines but they are not aware of their foolishness. When they get ill they look for medicine when it is too late. They do not know

[3]The four components are: body, breath, incorporeal and corporeal souls symbolised respectively by water, fire, wood and metal. See note 3 on page 36.

[4]The five elements of metal, wood, water, fire and earth. See also note 2 on page 36.

[5]The two divisions of one vitality: the positive yang and negative yin. See also note 5 on page 36.

that illnesses are caused by excess of food, drink and pleasures. They do not realise that inner ailments are latent in their bodies and when the latter manifest it is (sometimes) difficult to cure them.

Therefore, even before illnesses appear, you should use slow and quick fires to destroy their roots. For in your daily activities, your feelings of pleasure, anger, sorrow and joy are the causes of sickness, of pleasure affecting the heart, anger the liver, sorrow the incorporeal soul and joy the corporeal soul, thus injuring all the viscera. Do not neglect the roots of ailments because they seem to be slight and have not developed fully for when illnesses manifest you will have serious trouble. So before they appear they should be got rid of through the eyes;[6] how then can illness develop?

During the formation of the foetus in the mother's womb, in the first phase heaven begets the element of water in the pupils of the eyes which are linked with the kidneys; in the second phase earth produces the element of fire in the corners of the eyes which are linked with the heart; in the third phase heaven creates the element of wood in the irises which are linked with the liver; in the fourth phase earth produces the element of metal in the whites of the eyes which are linked with the lungs; and in the fifth phase heaven creates the element of earth in the upper and lower eyelids which are linked with the stomach. Thus the essences of all five viscera are in the eyes whereas original spirit, although seated in the brain, also manifests through the organs of seeing.

The whole body is negative except the two eyes which are positive. It is due to this small amount of positive yang in the eyes that man is not overwhelmed by the negative yin. This positive yang should be used at the beginning of alchemical

[6]The use of quick and slow fires transforms impurities in the body into tears.

training to root out all latent ailments that have accumulated in the body.

Quick fire is used to shift spirit's fire into the stove (under the navel) and was called 'shifting fire' by the ancients. By 'shifting' is meant arousing the inner fire so that both outer and inner fires act on each other in order to enlarge all obstructed psychic channels and clear them of obstructions. Since positive fire is stronger than generative force, it drives the latter into all parts of the body to remove all impurities thus preventing the development of ailments.

You can use the hypnotist's crystal ball (or any round object) for your practice in the morning and evening. First sit in meditative posture until your mind is settled and then place a crystal ball in front of you in such a position that it is neither too close nor too far and neither too high nor too low but in line with the spot between the eyes. After gazing at the ball for some time tears will flow; they are saline and smelly and are the residue of (inner) combustion similar to tears caused by feelings and emotions such as sadness, etc. After employing this 'shifting fire' to remove latent ailments, you should immediately use slow fire to soothe the pupils which otherwise may be injured by the heat. For slow fire helps the psychic channels that have dilated to shrink so that the breath that has spread to all parts in the body can return to its former position (under the navel). This slow fire is called 'calming fire' whose characteristic is immobilisation. You should use it by closing your eyes completely and concentrating on the spot between them in order to drive the breath back to the lower tan t'ien (under the navel). This concentration should last until the concept of the self and others is completely wiped out and body and mind no longer exist; only then can your concentration be effective. (While doing this) your tongue should plug the heavenly pool in the palate. In time the sweet dew which tastes like honey will go down (the jen mo channel in) the throat until it reaches the lower tan t'ien cavity where it changes into negative generative force which then descends to the testicles where it creates spermatozoa.

Therefore, pure saliva is the most precious thing that preserves our physical strength and calls for special care. When saliva is adequate the element of water is full in the lower abdomen causing the eyes to gleam with the pupils and whites well defined. When ailments are latent in the body the pupils are not clear and the whites of the eyes contain red or yellow streaks. You should then begin your practice until your eyes are like those of a healthy child whose pupils are bright and surrounded by a bluish white; only then are you free from latent ailments.

Physiology says that the eyes appear first when the foetus is being formed and the pupils twelve days later. Anatomy tells us that tears come from a fluid which washes the eyeballs; and that below the nasal cavity is a duct which discharges tears and snivel and is linked with the viscera in the body. It is by this duct that (latent) inner ailments are expelled for there is no other channel for the purpose.

The time set for employing quick and slow fires should be in the proportion of three to seven in order to avoid ill-effects from indiscriminate use.

After receiving instruction from my masters Liao Jan and Liao K'ung I gazed at a lighted incense stick which I later replaced with a crystal ball to arouse quick fire; and closed my eyes to make pointed concentration to kindle the slow fire in order to lower the (vital) breath in my heart to stabilise my spirit and intellect. As a result my ears heard no sounds and my breath became like a very fine thread that seemed not to be but was there until all my thoughts ceased and all my feelings and emotions came to an end. Then the element of fire in my heart went down while the waterly element in my lower abdomen soared up spontaneously. With the tip of my tongue touching the palate the two glands secreted plentiful saliva and my mouth was soon full of it; it was sweet like honey and went down at one gulp causing my lower abdomen to vibrate strongly. Suddenly my mind and intellect became still and void and first my four limbs and then the whole body disappeared without leaving any trace of myself. Like something that after reaching its limit turns round this utter stillness was followed by motion and all of a sudden the vital force vibrated strongly causing my penis to stand erect, which proved that real fire which had remained dormant for some time had begun to move itself.

Question All Taoist books mention the alchemical agent without teaching about fire. Will you please explain the 'phases of fire' (huo hou) so that future students will not be confused about them?

Answer 'Phases of fire' is a general term. 'Fire' is the inner heat and 'phases' are the six stages of purification by fire. The word 'fire' here has eighteen meanings which agree with the orderly stages of purification; hence the role played by it in each stage is different. If you do not receive instruction from an enlightened master you will never be clear about all this. The phases of fire, that is the stages of purification by fire and the production of the alchemical agent are in sequence and should not be mixed up. This is like making a brick; clay is first mixed with water and then baked by fire so that it becomes a brick. If a brick is not baked by fire it will turn to mud in the rain. Likewise the alchemical agent can be gathered only after (the generative force has been) purified by fire; only then can it produce the golden elixir, otherwise it will decay.

The Feng Huo Ching says: 'When the text uses terms such as *kindling the fire, leading it, forcing the fire with fire* and *stopping it* they all mean the fire kindled by breathing.

'When it mentions terms such as: *freeing the fire, driving it (into), lowering it, shifting fire, calming fire, fire in its own house* and *the heart's fire,* they all mean fire derived from spirit.

'When it uses terms such as: *Circulating the fire, gathering it, lifting it, fire in the house of water, negative fire, fire immersed in water, and fire in the stove,* they all mean fire derived from prenatal vitality.

'Fire kindled by breathing transforms the generative fluid derived from the digestion of food, into generative force. Fire derived from spirit transforms the generative force into vitality. Fire derived from (prenatal) vitality purifies breathing and contributes to the manifestation of spirit. Spiritual fire sublimates spirit which will return to the state of nothingness. Thus from start to finish the successful practice of immortality is by means of fire.'

Therefore, without explanation by an enlightened master it is very difficult to understand these eighteen phases of fire.

Question Will the old master explain these eighteen phases one by one?

Answer 'Kindling the fire' is by breathing through the nose which comprises an inhalation and an exhalation during which the small drug (hsiao yo or microcosmic alchemical agent) is produced and gathered. The air that goes down and up in the body is called the 'gentle breeze' (sun feng). As each breath enters the body your concentration (causes the generative force) to rise (in the tu mo channel in the spine) from the mortal cavity (at the root of the penis) to the head, and as the following exhalation leaves the body your concentration causes (the generative force) to descend (in the jen mo channel) from the head back to the mortal cavity. This is your concentration that turns the wheel of the law (i.e. the microcosmic orbiting).

The fire kindled by breathing, although originally tangible, should be treated as intangible (i.e. disregarded) for if you cling to it it will become harmful. To be effective it should be regarded as non-existent yet existing; in this propitious condition the generative force is bound to return to the lower tan t'ien (under the navel).[7]

The mechanism of the rise and fall (of the generative force in the microcosmic orbit) is called 'closing and opening' (ho p'i)[8] and also 'a flute without holes' which is 'played in reverse'.[9]

In the absence of stirring thought when the penis stands erect, the practiser should breathe in outer air which reaching the mortal cavity (at the base of the penis) causes the (negative) vital breath there to rise (in the jen mo channel) to the centre of vitality (the lower tan t'ien under the navel). After this he should breathe out so that the (negative) vital breath in

[7]Most practisers fail in their training because they do not know how to control this fire which intensifies the very passions which they intend to cut off. Hence many religious men break the rules of pure living and commit immoral acts which can be easily avoided by the ordinary man.

[8]*Closing* (ho) *opening* (p'i) are two Taoist terms. When outer air is breathed in it reaches the lower abdomen and pushes up the vital force; this is *closing* the mechanism of breathing so that the air goes down while inner vitality goes up to the head. When breathing out, outer air is expelled from the lower abdomen while the vital force, now free from pressure, returns to the lower abdomen; this is *opening* the mechanism of breathing so that outer air is rejected while inner vitality goes down.

[9]Readers should not confound this Taoist term with the ch'an (zen) idiom of a 'flute without holes' which is the mind closed to all sense data and whose melody can be understood and enjoyed by enlightened people. He who has acquired 'a flute without holes' understands the Mind Dharma as presented in the three volumes of our Ch'an and Zen Teaching series, Rider, London.

the chiang kung centre (the solar plexus) descends to the lower tan t'ien. After repeating this exercise several times, the penis will shrink back to normal and the practiser will feel very comfortable.

Therefore, each in and out breath shakes the field of the elixir (the lower tan t'ien under the navel) which is linked with the testicles by the genital duct (ch'un hsien)[10] by which the negative generative force reaches them to change into semen. This liquid contains spermatozoa; if it follows its earthly course it will flow out to produce offspring; but if it reverses this course it will contribute to the production of the golden elixir. This is only a matter of following or reversing the way of the world, which the ordinary man cannot understand. So it is imperative that you call on enlightened masters in order not to spoil your future.

Question What do you mean by 'leading the fire'?

Answer When you breathe in and out your concentration causes the generative force to rise and fall (in the microcosmic orbit) thus slowly turning the wheel of the law. Count from one to ten and then from ten to a hundred breaths with the heart (mind) following the counting to prevent it from wandering outside. When the heart and breathing are in unison, this is called *'locking up the monkey heart'* and *'tying up the running horse of intellect'*. The Tan Ching says:

> Let all thought come and go; awareness
> Of them without clinging is true training.
> All attachments are wrong whereas
> Inertness to false voidness leads.

[10]The genital duct runs from the testicles through the mortal gate at the base of the penis to the genital gate at the tip of the penis.

Mindfulness should give way to mindlessness so that the heart (the seat of nature) is empty (of all stirrings), becomes incorporeal and spiritual and beyond birth and death. If you want to get rid of wrong thoughts you should hold on to correct awareness and they will cease of themselves so that your heart will be like the bright moon in space, immaculate and containing no foreign matter. As the heart gets used to this condition it will be free from all illusions culminating in the death of the heart and resurrection of the spirit. For if spirit is not settled the light of (essential) nature does not manifest and if intellect is not frozen passions cannot be cut off. In this state of serenity when the inmost vibrates of itself you should immediately take advantage of its vibration to gather the microcosmic alchemical agent. This is called 'leading the fire' (to gather the agent).

Question Each in and out breath causes the ascent and descent (of vital breath). You have spoken of 'blocking breath' and now mention 'the leading of fire'. I am not clear and pray you to explain all this fully.

Answer This is because you misunderstand my instruction. At the start the first ascent and descent (of vital breath) that turn the wheel of the law, serve to identify the thinking process with the turning wheel in order to stop all wandering thoughts. Then the following inhalation and exhalation which send the (vital) breath up and down to complete a full orbit thereby stopping the arousal of the genital organ, is to block the drain of generative fluid; but this should only be done after the alchemical agent has been gathered. Please ponder over all this carefully. These two kinds of breathing are motivated by the sole thought of 'leading the inner fire' to turn the wheel of the law (for the double purpose of stopping all wandering thoughts and of blocking the drain of generative fluid).

Question What do you mean by 'stopping the fire'?

Answer By 'stopping the fire' is meant discontinuing all alchemical breathing.[11]

Question Why is the alchemical breathing discontinued?

Answer When the lower abdomen is full of generative force the inner fire is stopped by discontinuing all (alchemical) breathing through the nose. The patriarch Cheng Yang said: 'When the alchemical agent ripens the use of fire should be stopped for continual fire will spoil it.' The immortal Ch'ung Hsu said: 'Only when the time to stop the fire comes can the macrocosmic alchemical agent be gathered for the breakthrough.'

The time to stop the fire comes after the golden light has manifested twice; it is the time to gather the (macrocosmic alchemical) agent by discontinuing all (alchemical) breathing through the nose. If the practiser waits until the third manifestation of the golden light to stop the fire he will miss the mark and the macrocosmic alchemical agent will be spoilt.

Fire should be stopped before gathering the macrocosmic agent for the breakthrough. After the second manifestation of the golden light the agent should be gathered to restore fully the generative force, vitality and spirit. If breathing through the nose is used at the time of gathering the agent, the latter is bound to scatter at night for the air breathed in and out can shake and spoil the generative and vital forces. Hence the discontinuing of all (alchemical) breathing through the nose to stop the fire.

---

[11]Although the practiser continues breathing as usual he should not use in and out breaths to arouse the inner fire which will then cease of itself.

Question If in and out breathing is not used (alchemically) how can the generative and vital forces go up and down (in the microcosmic orbit)?

Answer Although breathing through the nose is not used (alchemically) the inner (vital) breath (in the body) is pushed up and down by the practiser's concentration. So each ascent and descent of the (vital) breath accord with his will and turn the wheel of the law; only this can be called 'stopping the fire' to gather the alchemical agent.

Question What do you mean by 'forcing the fire with fire'?

Answer It means using in and out breaths to gather the alchemical agent. Driving the generative and vital forces into the stove (in the lower abdomen) by means of the gentle breeze (breathing) is to check the generative force and is called 'forcing the fire with fire'.

The element of fire in the generative force, vitality and spirit *moves* from A to D (for cleansing) and then to G where it *stays* for a while, and is called the ascending positive fire; it subsequently *re-starts* from G down to J (for purification) and then *stops* at A and is called the descending negative fire. Thus its *move* (hsin), *stay* (chu), *restart* (chi) and *stop* (chih) are the four phases of the alchemical process which includes both cleansing and purification. Practisers should ponder over all this and become aware of the mechanism.

Each rotation from A to D, G, J (and back to A) includes the ascent of positive yang and descent of negative yin, the shutting and opening of the mechanism of breathing, the use of the bellows, the six phases of orbiting and the gathering and purification of the alchemical agent. The practiser's understanding depends on whether or not he has met an enlightened master.

If you have not met an experienced teacher but rely on your own intellect to understand the Taoist scriptures, and if during the ascent of positive fire you merely count (9 x 4 = 36 x 5 phases from A to B, C, E and F) 180 times and during the descent of its negative counterpart (6 x 4 = 24 x 5 phases from G, to H, I, K, L) 120 times without knowing the shutting and opening of the mechanism of breathing, and the six phases of alchemical process which complete the efficient working of the microcosmic orbit, you will fail in your practice of 'forcing the fire with fire' and all your efforts will be sterile.

(Above are the four kinds of fire kindled by breathing).

Question The Feng Huo Ching lists another seven kinds of fire; what does the 'freezing of fire' mean?

Answer 'Freezing the fire' is freezing and driving spirit into the cavity of vitality (under the navel). The Tan Ching says: 'All masters taught only the freezing (or fixing) of spirit in the cavity of vitality.'

To fix spirit consists of concentration which draws the pupils of both eyes as close as possible to each other. This is called 'freezing the spirit', 'looking backward' and 'uniting the sun with the moon' for the purpose of returning to the prenatal state in which, while in the mother's womb, the two eyes of the foetus are in unison, and nature and life are one. At birth nature and life divide in two and are thus separated.

'Freezing the fire' means that both eyes in unison look down into the cavity of vitality (the lower tan t'ien under the navel) which is called the gate to life (ming men) which is below and behind the navel and below and before the kidneys, the distance between it and the front and rear of the abdomen being in the proportion of seven to three. It hangs under and between the kidneys below and is linked with the ni wan or

brain above and the soles of the feet below, being the source of
prenatal Tao (immortality). Hence it is said: 'This cavity is not
material and is the union of both the male (chien) and female
(k'un) principles; it is called the cavity of spiritual vitality
which contains both the elements of fire and water in the
generative force. The ancient medical science calls it the 'gate
to life' and the Taoists call it the 'cavity of vitality'. My master
Liao K'ung said: 'When blood reaches this cavity (under the
navel) it changes into negative generative force which finds its
way into the testicles.'

All students should know that, in order to fix (and drive)
spirit into the cavity of vitality, a serious practiser should sit in
meditation in a quiet room, turn back his eyes to look into this
cavity, with only awareness of but no clinging to it, that is he
first feels its presence and then forgets about it. While fixing
spirit his mind should be empty (of sense data) with attachment to neither form nor relative voidness in order to preserve
its radiant stillness and clear immateriality. At this stage only
the breathing is felt with inner harmony between the upper
and lower parts of his body the outcome of which is an
ineffable comfort. Suddenly his eyes (seem to) fall from his
face into that cavity (of the lower tan t'ien under the navel)
causing him to feel that his body no longer exists and that true
vitality fills the abode of spirit which will hold it.

Question What do you mean by 'driving the fire'?

Answer It is the positive fire as will be explained in Chapter 6.
Chapter 4 has already dealt with gathering the microcosmic
outer alchemical agent in order to return it to the stove (in the
lower abdomen); since this agent is still not yet sublimated by
fire, it can drain away like tea poured continuously into a cup
which overflows and spreads outside. This positive fire can
transmute the agent in the stove into vitality (in order to stop

its overflow). This stage is much more important than merely gathering the agent as explained in Chapter 4.

After gathering and holding the outer alchemical agent as previously explained, the practiser, while sitting in meditation, should now close his eyes, roll them from left to right nine times and pause to see if the inner circle of light has opened its gate. If it does not he should wait a little and then close his eyes to make the same nine turns for a second time and pause to see if the light manifests between them and opens its gate. If it does not he should continue making the same number of turns for a third and fourth time. He thus makes the same number of turns four times. This is 'driving the fire' for the ascent of positive fire.

Question What do you mean by 'lowering the fire'?

Answer 'Lowering the fire' is making it retreat. The Tan Ching says: 'The ascent of positive fire is by thirty-six turns and the descent of its negative counterpart is by twenty-four turns.'

In the descent of negative fire to open the gate, the practiser should roll his eyes from G backward to D, A and J six times. He should then close his eyes to look at the inner circle of light. Seeing that the gate is still unopen he should do this four times. This is the descent of fire.

Only the eyes are positive whereas the rest of the body is negative. It is these positive eyes which will overcome the whole negative body so that gradually the positive principle (yang) will develop daily while the negative principle (yin) will decrease correspondingly. As time passes the whole body will become positive. This is what the saying means by: 'If the negative principle is not entirely wiped out immortality cannot be achieved.' This also is the retreat of negative fire.

The term 'shifting fire' has been explained earlier (see page 50). 'Shifting' is motionless change, that is transmutation by quick fire which results in nothing any longer having form or shape whether seen closely or from a distance, and includes the elimination of every impure residue. Only this can be called true efficiency.

The term 'calming fire' means immobilisation (see page 50) with no idea of the self and others in order to ensure the emptiness of both body and intellect; then all of a sudden the practiser feels as if he comes out of his physical body to look at his original face. Only this can be called real achievement.

Question What do you mean by 'fire in li' (i.e. fire in the house of fire)?

Answer The heart is the house of fire. When the heart is stirred the penis stands erect in spite of the absence of thoughts. This is real fire in its house, which arouses the genital organ, and although thoughts are absent, this fire is not the genuine one which vibrates at the living hour of tsu (between 11 p.m. and 1 a.m.) when the penis erects.[12] If you gather the alchemical agent at this unsuitable moment it is too young because vitality is not full and can scatter easily; hence the agent should not be gathered for it is not the proper time to do so. Only when the penis stands erect at the living hour of tsu can the agent be gathered, and this should be done quickly for this is the proper time, but if you wait until this moment has passed to pick up the agent, the latter has grown old (and is useless) because vitality has scattered after the passing of fire in its own house.

Question What is the heart's fire?

Answer When the eyes twinkle and the heart vibrates in sympathy, this is the 'chief fire' (chun huo), also called the

[12]See note 4 on page 12 for full explanation of the hour of tsu.

heart's fire. It is evil fire aroused by thoughts and should be avoided by the practiser.

When the eyes see the opposite sex thereby giving rise to (evil) thoughts, the heart moves in sympathy and arouses the genital organ, if the practiser then tries to gather the alchemical agent, the impure generative fluid will produce an illusory agent. This illusory agent is likened to a football which, being kicked continuously, will lose air and shrink. Likewise as thoughts increase the evil fire which becomes more intense, the genital organ will be aroused more frequently. If you wrongly think that the alchemical agent is being produced and strive to gather it, your efforts will be sterile, and you will only harm yourself. Your body seems to be strong (so long as this evil fire lasts) but your health suffers from the consequences and will really decline. Frequent arousal of sexual desire is likened to putting straw on the head while going to extinguish a big fire; you will only injure your body, and will not only fail to achieve immortality but will also run the risk of shortening your life.

Therefore, you should avoid gathering the alchemical agent when your heart's fire is aroused by evil thoughts.

The above seven kinds of fire: freezing, driving and lowering the fire, shifting fire, calming fire, fire in its own house and the heart's fire, come from spirit and can transmute the generative force into vitality. This spirit's fire derives from the spiritual power in the eyes, and if supported by postnatal breathing through the nostrils, can sublimate the generative force and sustain the inner vital breath.

My master Liao K'ung said: 'The generative force can be fully sublimated within a hundred days and will then fill the lower abdomen.'

This does not mean merely replacing the dissipated generative force as that force should be retained and developed so that you can recover the supply which was latent in you at the time of puberty. The fullness of prenatal vitality in your body is revealed by your genital organ which retracts (during the training).

The restoration of a full supply of generative and vital forces is by means of another seven kinds of fire which are: circulating the fire, gathering it, lifting it, fire in the house of water, negative fire, fire immersed in water and fire in the stove. These seven fires derive from prenatal vitality and contribute to the sublimation of in and out breaths for the manifestation of original spirit. By original spirit is meant that spirit of no spirit (which is inexpressible).

Question What do you mean by 'circulating the fire'?

Answer When the generative and vital forces vibrate you should use the mechanism of the bellows, the closing and opening method of breathing, the six phases of the alchemical process and the positive ascent and negative descent to circulate true fire raising it (to the brain) through the first gate at the base of the spine, the second gate between the kidneys and the third gate in the occiput. All three gates are opened by an inhalation. The following exhalation sends the fire down from the original cavity of spirit (tsu ch'iao in the brain) to the chiang kung centre (at the solar plexus) and then back to the cavity of vitality (under the navel). Thus a full breath comprises an ascent and a descent of true fire; this is circulating the fire.

Question What do you mean by 'gathering the fire'?

Answer 'Gathering' means collecting (the fire). The ancients spoke of the alchemical agent without mentioning the fire which is the generative and vital forces. Fire is also the alchemical agent. So when true fire vibrates you should collect it.

If you cultivate only (essential) nature and disregard (eternal) life your practice is incomplete and inefficient. For the cultivation of nature alone ensures only the descent of positive fire without the ascent of (vital) breath from below; the result will be that nature and life cannot unite. Therefore, you should gather fire to lift up the (vital) breath below.

Question What do you mean by 'lifting the fire'?

Answer After fire has been gathered it tends to develop; you should lift it through the three gates in the backbone up to the ni wan or brain and then lower it (in the jen mo or channel of function) to the chiang kung cavity (the solar plexus) before returning it to the centre of vitality (under the navel); in so doing you should use your non-discriminative concentration to lift and lower it in order to complete a full orbit.

Hun Jan Tsu said: 'When vitality manifests it vibrates strongly and fire develops under the navel; this is the moment when you should lift it up to invigorate your body which has been weakened by the drain of generative force. The latter will in time be fully recovered to lengthen your life.'

Question What do you mean by 'fire in k'an (the house of water)'?

Answer K'an and li[13] stand for the lower abdomen and heart respectively. Vitality and spirit are respective functionings of k'an and li. Spirit in li (the house of fire) is (essential) nature and vitality in k'an (the house of water) is (eternal life.)

Fire in the house of water stands for vitality in vibration which then forms a (kind of) bellows (extending) from 1.2

[13]K'an and li are two diagrams symbolising water and fire respectively according to the Book of Change.

inches below the heart to 1.3 inches under the navel, which is linked through the mortal cavity (sheng szu ch'iao at the root of the penis) with the genital gate (yang kuan at the tip of the penis). This is 'fire in the house of water'.

Question What do you mean by 'negative fire' (kun huo)?

Answer Kun stands for the lower tan t'ien (under the navel), also called the stove. Huo is vitality which takes advantage of the fire in the house of water to descend into the channel of control (tu mo in the spine) wherein ventilation provided by in and out breathing transmutes the generative force into the alchemical agent in order to carry it up (in the microcosmic orbit). For the positive yang cannot accumulate without aid from the negative yin; hence vitality should join the generative force to become fire. This is the union of positive (vitality) with negative (generative force) which will then ascend to the head (through the tu mo or channel of control). If evil thoughts arise at this stage neither the generative nor vital forces can be put into the right orbit but will enter the urethra causing aching inflammation there with fever which will cease only after a reddish yellow urine has been discharged. This is the harmful effect of stirring thoughts at this stage. If the generative and vital forces pass through the mortal cavity (at the base of the penis) they will enter two channels in the thighs which will be obstructed by an accumulation of generative fluid.

Question What do you mean by 'fire immersed in water'?

Answer When the generative and vital forces are in their cavity (under the navel) they are fire but when they leave it (to drain away) they take a liquid form. To gather the alchemical agent is to hold vitality in its cavity which is called the cavity of true vitality (chen ch'i hsueh) or lower tan t'ien which is where true vitality manifests and which is linked with the genital organ. The generative force is watery and heavy and tends to sink whereas spirit is fiery and light and tends to soar. Man is usually unaware of the flow of vitality and is thereby subject to birth, old age, illness and death. The vital force that scatters is not the air breathed in and out but true vitality that sustains the generative force. Whether a man lives or dies depends solely on the presence or absence of vitality. Death is caused by the exhaustion of vitality and although a dead body remains the same as when alive, it only lacks vitality.

Question You have spoken of vitality which drains away continuously; how does one stop its drain?

Answer The only method is to shut the genital gate (yang kuan) in order to ensure long life free from death.

The treatise Ching Hsien Lun says: 'He whose genital gate is closed enjoys long life.' All students should seek instruction from enlightened masters and strive to hold both water and fire in the same cavity (i.e. the lower tan t'ien under the navel). Water is below and fire is above. When fire is immersed in water, it will stop soaring up thereby causing the heart to be empty (i.e. not to stir); and as water is scorched by fire, it will stop flowing down. This is water and fire in stable equilibrium (shui huo chi chi) which will in time produce vitality. When the penis stands erect of itself, this is due to the generative and vital forces developing in their cavity (the lower tan t'ien under the navel) and is called fire manifesting in water.

My master said: 'When the generative and vital forces in the lower tan t'ien cavity move away they become liquid but when they return to that cavity they are prenatal vitality.' Therefore, each time you notice the manifestation of fire in water, you should immediately turn it back to the lower tan t'ien cavity in order to sublimate it. Only when six unusual states manifest can you be certain that the immortal seed is being completely formed.

Question What do you mean by 'fire in the stove'?

Answer When spirit and vitality vibrate in the lower tan t'ien cavity (under the navel), the latter is called the *stove* and when they rise to the upper tan t'ien (in the brain) the latter is called the *cauldron*. In the absence of spirit and vitality neither stove nor cauldron can be spoken of.[14]

Hence the old patriarch Ch'ung Hsu Tsu said: 'The cauldron is originally non-existent.' The patriarch Lu Tsu said: 'Only those who know what stove, cauldron and bellows really are can use them effectively.' To produce real 'fire in the stove' requires authentic instruction from enlightened masters in order to know how to gather the outer drug (outer alchemical agent).

We now discuss all this in detail for the benefit of students who should know the correct method of practice. As to the gathering of the outer (alchemical) agent, the practiser whose penis is erect, should ascertain whether or not it is at the living hour of tsu (between 11 p.m. and 1 a.m.). If so he should immediately block the genital gate (yang kuan above the genital organ) to collect the alchemical agent until he is fully aware of success.

If the generative and vital forces burst out causing the body to bend a little, the practiser should press his middle finger on the mortal gate (to stop the emission) and

---

[14]As in the case of ignorant worldlings who let the generative and vital forces drain away in their quest of sexual pleasures.

immediately set in motion the mechanism of the gentle breeze, the six phases of alchemical purification, the bellows and the closing and opening process of breathing to drive back and gather (the generative and vital forces). In order to avoid eventual leakage, in and out breaths are used to seal up the two forces. After bringing them under control, they should be immediately put into microcosmic orbit for sublimation by fire, during which the generative force will be transformed into vitality. This is the gradual method of transmuting the generative force into vitality. When both generative and vital forces are fully restored, the practiser's body will not differ from that of a youth at puberty.

The Ts'ui Hsu P'ien says:

When the bright moon from the south-west shines on the
road
Immortality unfolds its endless path.

This is the lower tan t'ien cavity (under the navel) full of the alchemical agent which reveals to the eyes the beauty of positive vital breath. Wherever the practiser walks, stays, sits or reclines, he will see a white light in front of him, and, as time passes, this white light changes into a golden one. This is the first manifestation of the golden light, and when it appears for a second time, the practiser should stop the fire. The least carelessness on his part at this stage will cause risk and peril leading to utter failure; this is the most difficult phase.

The above seven kinds of fire come from prenatal vitality and can sublimate all in and out breaths in order to contribute to the manifestation of original spirit. This original spirit is the spirit of no spirit which can use spiritual fire to destroy its (physical) form to return to nothingness in order to achieve immortality. This spiritual fire is the spirit's golden light that then appears. Students should seek authentic instructions from enlightened masters in order to realise this spiritual fire of the golden light and finally join the rank of golden immortals.

If you think you realise that golden light when many (tiny) golden sparks appear in your eyes you are utterly wrong. For this golden light manifests in front of you while your essential body (fa shen) in the great emptiness gradually comes closer to it. When the light of this body joins and mingles with the golden light (in front of you) you will realise your essential body which will then enter your physical body; the latter will absorb that spiritual body and in three years' time will be sublimated into pure vitality. This is the manifestation of positive spirit (yang shen) which will take form when it gathers in one place or will become pure vitality when it scatters to fill the great emptiness which will be its boundless body.

I received instructions from my masters Liao Jen and Liao K'ung and also called on over thirty old teachers but only P'eng Mow Ch'ang, Ch'iao Ch'iao, T'an Chi Ming and my two teachers knew the secrets of the twin cultivation of (essential) nature and (eternal) life. I now divulge these secrets to sincere students so that when they meet their teachers they should ascertain if the latter can reply satisfactorily to the questions answered in this book. I urge them not to believe in heretics and imposters who know nothing about alchemy but pose as competent masters; their so-called teachings have nothing to do with the doctrine of the cultivation of (essential) nature and (eternal) life because their sole aim is to make a living and so they deceive and mislead their pupils who will pass their lifetime aimlessly without achieving any results.

6

GATHERING THE MICROCOSMIC INNER ALCHEMICAL AGENT[1]

The method of gathering the microcosmic inner alchemical agent consists of rolling the eyes from left to right and vice versa to raise and lower the inner fire. The meditator should first direct his eyes down and roll them from the left up to the top of the head, thence lowering them to the right to look into the navel and the centre of vitality below it to complete a full turn as indicated in the diagram by the sun held in his left hand which rises from A to D and G and then sinks from G to J. This movement should be repeated thirty-six times for the ascent *positive fire* to open the mysterious gate (see page 73). After this he should roll his eyes from G to D, A and J as indicated by the moon held in his right hand. This movement should be repeated twenty-four times for the descent of *negative fire*.

Chapter 4 has dealt with gathering the (microcosmic) outer alchemical agent to restore the generative force and invigorate the brain. It consists of raising the positive fire (in the tu mo or channel of control) to the head thirty-six times in its advance called the ascent of positive fire, and then lower it

[1]See note 3 on page xv (Preface).

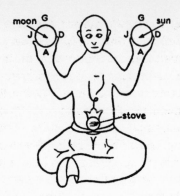

Figure 5 This symbolic diagram is copied from the original text. It means that the meditator should squint as indicated while his hands are placed on the legs and close to the lower abdomen in the usual meditation posture.

(in the channel of function or jen mo in the front of the body) twenty-four times in its retreat called the descent of negative fire. Each rotation is completed in a full (in and out) breath during which spirit and vitality move or halt together in the juxtaposed orbits of the earth (i.e. the lower abdomen) and the sun (the head), spirit being set in motion by the (movements of the eyes), and vitality by the combined action of vital and generative forces already gathered. These movements and halts concern the gathering of the (microcosmic) outer alchemical agent which frees the body from ailments whereas the (microcosmic) inner alchemical agent preserves (perma-nent) life which is prenatal vitality.

This chapter discusses the method of using the micro-cosmic inner fire that passes through sublimating phases at the cardinal points D and J (see *figure 2* on page 15) to produce the (microcosmic) inner alchemical agent, which method is also called 'inner copulation' (nei chiao kou) meaning that after you have gathered enough of the (microcosmic) outer alchemical agent, true vitality, driven by ventilation and fire, will soar up to the brain; you should then roll your eyes from left to right in a complete circle in order to push vitality up and down so that the vital breath in the brain unites with the nervous system. At this stage the brain will develop fully and a bright light will manifest (between the eyes); you should now gather the (microcosmic) inner alchemical agent; this is commonly called the preparation of the golden elixir. This bright light is the mysterious gate (hsuan kuan) about which it is said:

> Your mouth cannot explain what appears before you;
> Seeing it you will be relieved of all concern.

My master said: 'Roll round the positive yang and negative yin (i.e. the two eyes) to shake the brain in order to pull out from its centre spirit which has developed and will then emerge from the mysterious gate (i.e. the bright light that has manifested).'

Ch'en Ni Wan said: 'The real positive yang and negative yin are true Tao (immortality) which is right in front of you and should not be sought elsewhere.'

The Huo Hou Ko says: 'To reach the mysterious gate requires solitary vigilance the secret of which lies in the eyes.'

Ch'ien Feng Lao Jen said: 'The sun and the moon,[2] when turning round, unite the positive yang with the negative yin so that a glorious light emerges from the centre of the brain. If you only gather the (microcosmic) outer alchemical agent during the "inner copulation" of the male and female principles and do not gather the (microcosmic) inner alchemical agent during the phases at D and J (in the orbit)

---

[2]The left and right eyes stand respectively for the sun and the moon, i.e. the positive yang and negative yin.

you are like a cart without wheels or a boat without rudders.'
How then can you achieve your goal?

Moreover when the (microcosmic) outer alchemical
agent has been returned to the stove (under the navel) if
positive and negative fires are not sent up and down (the
psychic channels) through the various phases of sublimation
in the microcosmic orbit, the generative and vital forces cannot
be transmuted into the wondrous light, that glory of the golden
elixir which makes the practiser springtime fresh, his blood
circulate freely, his breathing unobstructed and his digestion
easy. If the (microcosmic) outer alchemical agent is left intact
in the stove (under the navel) it cannot be transformed into
vitality by fire; you will then find it hard to restore your original
(prenatal) body which cannot leak and is most precious. (This
is because) the continual drain of generative fluid empties the
testicles (of energy), just as a full vessel overflows when more
water is added if there is no fire to turn that water into steam.
Therefore, the generative fluid, when full, will be discharged
sooner or later as proved by nocturnal emission. Without an
experienced master to teach you it will be very difficult to
understand alchemy, and in spite of your efforts you will not
be able to stop the discharge of generative fluid. Is this not
most regrettable?

Question You have said that after gathering the (microcosmic)
outer alchemical agent, the practiser will fail to transmute the
generative force into vitality if he does not raise the positive fire
and lower its negative counterpart; and that he will not be able
to stop the drain of the elixir at night. I have several times
succeeded in producing and gathering the (microcosmic)
outer alchemical agent and in spite of my making no use of
these ascents and descents, I never had nocturnal emissions.
What is the reason?

Answer Your question is most welcome. As you have said, you have only begun to fill your testicles; later on when they are full, if you do not raise and lower the fire, this is like making bricks without baking them so that they are hard and resistant; they will turn to mud again when exposed to rain. Therefore, these ascents and descents are indispensable (for they play the same role as the fire that bakes bricks). This is what the Tan Ching means by: 'If the cauldron is devoid of true seed, it is like boiling an empty vessel (which will be damaged).'

I now deal with all this in detail. Your two eyes, though separate, have only one root; if both eyes roll round their root will move as well. The left eye stands for the East whose element is wood and the right eye for the West whose element is metal. The element of wood turns westward to unite with the element of metal and the latter turns eastward to mingle with the former. This is the union of both elements causing the (vital) breath in the brain and the psychic strength to develop, expand and unite into one whole reaching the core of the brain where it transmutes the (microcosmic) outer alchemical agent (already gathered there) into life-preserving true vitality; this is (eternal) life returning to (essential) nature to become one whole; only thus can nature and life be worked on successfully.

The practiser would make a grave mistake if he sat motionless to cultivate (essential) nature while disregarding (eternal) life. For instance, the shell of an egg is likened to the body and the yolk to life. When a young chicken is hatched the shell is broken and abandoned, but if it is broken before incubation you cannot expect a young chicken to emerge from it. Therefore, a practiser of Tao should preserve his physical body with the same care as he would a precious gem. He should know that:

Without the body the Tao cannot be attained
But with the body Truth never can be realised.[3]

and when his training has been effective then it will be time to
leave the body.

True nature is prenatal vitality in its cell (ch'i pao) on the
top of the medulla oblongata. If vitality is allowed to pass
through the back of the head and down to the base of the spine
to drain away through the anus and genital organ, its
exhaustion will cause death.

This exhaustion of vitality is in no way related to the
breath that comes in and out through the nostrils and mouth.
In nocturnal emissions the generative fluid carries with it
(some) vitality which thus leaves its vibrating cell in the centre
of the brain to pass into the spine and then reach its base to
drain away. It is this vitality which animates spermatozoa
which, in its absence, become lifeless and non-reproductive.
This cell is linked with the brain above it, the base of the spine
below and the whole nervous system in the body and is the
source of the vital energy of life.

When the heart is stirred by sexual desires, it is
impossible to draw back this vital force which will drain down
in the marrow of the spine to leave the body; it will then be
impossible to cultivate (eternal) life. That which so drains off
is prenatal vitality and although sexual intercourse has not
actually occurred, it nevertheless runs away by the genital gate.

[3]The body should be preserved so that it can be used as a medium to achieve
immortality, but if you do not abandon it you will not realise the Truth.

7

HOLDING ON TO THE CENTRE TO REALISE THE ONENESS OF HEAVEN AND EARTH

To hold on to the centre to realise the oneness of heaven and earth is achieved only by uniting the sun and the moon. The sun stands for the heart and the moon for the lower tan t'ien cavity (under the navel), respectively symbolised by the dragon (the female or negative vitality) and the tiger (the male or positive vitality).

When oneness of heaven and earth is achieved and the lights of the sun and moon mingle in front of the original cavity of spirit (tsu ch'iao in the centre of the brain between and behind the eyes) this is the macrocosmic alchemical agent of One Reality. This is the place (between and behind the eyes) where the generative force, vitality and spirit unite, where heart and intellect are void and where there is neither the self nor others.

In front of the cavity of spirit (between and behind the eyes) true vitality looks like a (radiant) circle which is called the Supreme Ultimate (t'ai chi), the Golden Elixir (chin tan) and the Original Awareness (yuan chueh).

Hence the prenatal heaven and earth and postnatal heart and the lower tan t'ien or the field of the elixir (under the navel) are called the four yin-yang (szu ko yin yang, positive and negative principles).

Chapters 1 to 4 teach the preliminary steps and 5 to 8 the transmuting methods. For it is first necessary to restore the generative force in order to invigorate the brain for the purpose of sustaining (eternal) life. Hence this gradual training should be clear to the student before he starts training to master the creative power of heaven and earth thereby sowing the true seed (of immortality).

Shang Yang Tsu said: 'It is up to the student to seek competent teachers.' He cannot produce the alchemical agent

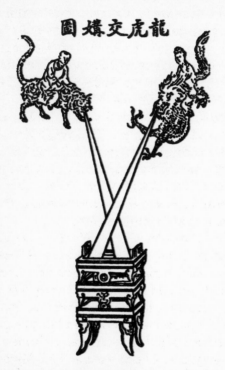

Figure 6 The dragon (negative vitality) and the tiger (positive vitality) 'copulating' in the alchemical cauldron in the brain to realise the oneness of heaven and earth.

by himself because if he is not well versed in the training he will not know what to do when encountering the mechanism of Creativity; this is due to his wrong assumption of knowing what he does not really know.

If he trains blindly without waiting for the mechanism of Creativity to manifest his practice will be not only futile but also very harmful. Readers are urged to be very careful on this point. It would be far better for him to wait until his face radiates before gathering the alchemical agent which he should then sublimate with fire in the microcosmic orbit in order to transmute it into vitality; when the generative force and vitality are full (essential) nature and (eternal) life will unite into one. For during each additional purification by microcosmic fire, the prenatal generative force, vitality and spirit will become one, and the practiser will be aware of the presence of the circle of light, somewhat similar to the bright sun in mid-heaven which appears in front of him. This results from successful practice of the first six steps (taught in Chapters 1 to 6) which purify the generative force in the body; this circle is called the Mysterious Gate (hsuan kuan). This Mysterious Gate is the most wonderful and profound cavity which is the Supreme Ultimate (t'ai chi) in the human body.

The Taoist Scriptures say: 'This cavity lies in the centre between heaven (head) and earth (lower abdomen) in the human body.' The patriarch Ch'iu Tsu said: 'It is wrong to seek it in the body and it is equally wrong to search for it outside. For when it manifests it becomes a cavity and when it does not it is undiscoverable.' The Hsin Ming Kuei Chih says: 'The Mysterious Cavity[1] is boundless; awareness of it, free from all clinging, is real achievement. This Mysterious Gate

[1] The Mysterious Gate and the Mysterious Cavity are the same thing; it is a gate when it appears in front of the practiser and is a cavity when it lies hidden in the body.

manifests in the condition of utter stillness but if a thought arises, it immediately slips into the postnatal realm and vanishes at once without leaving any trace. If it is further sought it cannot be found because of the clinging to form.'

My masters Liao Jan and Liao K'ung said: 'This Mysterious Gate is achieved by the practice of the first six steps (taught in Chapters 1 to 6). It manifests only when the generative force, vitality and spirit unite in the original cavity of spirit (tsu ch'iao between and behind the eyes) and is prenatal one vitality which forms a circle.'

My brother K'uei I Tsu said: 'When the generative force, vitality and spirit are full they soar up to cause the light of (essential) nature to manifest; this is the light of the vitality of One Reality.'

When bright stars and flashes of light are seen frequently they always herald the Mysterious Gate which is in space and manifests in front of the original cavity of spirit (between and behind the eyes); it is the real One Vitality, which is our 'original face', boundless like the great emptiness. Hence it is said: 'Prenatal One Vitality comes from nothingness.'

The practiser will see this Mysterious Gate (or circle of light) suddenly move away from him, and when it returns, he should gather and hold it first in the original cavity of spirit (between and behind the eyes) and then absorb it into the chiang kung centre (or solar plexus) where it will vibrate as revealed by a rare fragrance in his mouth. He should refrain from gathering the Mysterious Gate (by concentrating on it) immediately after its appearance because to do so will cause it to collide with and cause great pain to the brain, while self-inflicting troubles follow.

Great emptiness is that nebula which has settled and is called *Heavenly Oneness* (ch'ien i) in the Book of Change, *the All-pervading One* (i kuan) in Confucian classics, and *Holding*

on to One (shou i) in Taoist scriptures, all these terms meaning
the unity (of all things). The *all-pervading One* penetrates the
centre (of Reality in the brain i.e. the tsu chiao) and *Holding on
to One* upholds that centre. Hence after the basic vitality has
been absorbed in the abdomen, this is what the Tan Ching
means by: 'When One is realised nothing remains to be done.'

Question You have said the Mysterious Gate is like a circle and
that other philosophies teach the return to Oneness which is
also symbolised by a circle. Will you please explain their basic
theories, realisations and beneficial effects?

Answer This circle is achieved by the successful practice of the
first six steps (taught in Chapters 1 to 6). When prenatal
original vitality is realised the light of generative force, vitality
and spirit soars up and manifests in front of the original cavity
of spirit (tsu ch'iao between and behind the eyes). It is
indescribable and is expediently called Tao.

He who does not know the potency of the original cavity
of spirit cannot produce basic vitality. He who does not know
how the cauldron and stove work cannot produce this vitality.
He who does not know how to gather the alchemical agent,
cannot transmute the generative force into basic vitality and
lift it to the brain. He who does not know how to clear the eight
psychic channels, cannot circulate vitality through them. He
who does not know how to join up the four poles (i.e. prenatal
heaven and earth and postnatal heart and abdomen) cannot
gather this basic vitality. He who does not know how to raise
positive and lower negative fire, cannot develop the light of
basic vitality. When this prenatal basic vitality gathers to return
to its source it is expediently represented by a circle which is
prenatal true nature whose light emerges from the union of
generative force, vitality and spirit manifesting in front of the

original cavity of spirit (tsu ch'iao between and behind the eyes).

He who has this vitality lives and he who loses it dies. For the human body envelops vitality which in turn contains spirit. Hence when (vital) breath leaves the body a man dies and when vitality scatters, his spirit, lacking support, will become a ghost.

The circle (or Mysterious Gate) is achieved by successful practice of the seventh step (taught in this chapter) which consists of gathering basic vitality in order to hold on to the centre (between and behind the eyes) and realise the oneness (of things). He who succeeds in gathering it will see the light of (essential) nature appear and then scatter. Because of his successful practice of the method of uniting the sun with the moon and of the rise of vitality in front of the original cavity of spirit, this light will again appear and will in time disperse once more. He will see it appear again as clean and spotless as before) but since he fails to gather and hold it, it will again fly away. Thus he will miss it and so let the mechanism of Creativity slip away without achieving any results, which is most regrettable.

However, if he can unite the element of metal (male) with that of wood (female) and the sun with the moon in one place by drawing his pupils closely together in a squint and if he then concentrates them and looks within, he will see the light of true vitality appearing (between his eyes) in front of his original cavity of spirit which will then hold it to prevent it from running away; and the longer it is held the brighter it will be. When it becomes stable, it reveals the successful union of the dragon and tiger (i.e. the female and male vital breaths). When heart and lower abdomen are linked, heaven and earth are in perfect harmony; and when the dragon and tiger 'copulate', the positive and negative elements of earth unite, thus gathering the four symbols (szu hsiang, i.e. prenatal heaven and earth and postnatal heart and abdomen) in the central cavity (chung kung or the solar plexus) to produce the macrocosmic alchemical agent. The Book of Change calls this *the generative forces of heaven and earth* by means of which all things are reproduced without interruption.

The sexual union of man and woman begets offspring to continue the human race. The union of the positive and negative forces of heaven and earth creates myriads of things. Alchemy produces the macrocosmic agent by means of intercourse between the positive yang and negative yin.

If the macrocosmic alchemical agent is gathered when it is young it will disperse and there is no way to prevent this, but if the student has received instruction from an experienced master and knows the correct method he can gather and keep it in the cauldron (in the lower abdomen) to produce the golden nectar.

Question What is the macrocosmic alchemical agent and how can one transmute it into golden nectar and return the latter to the cauldron (in the lower abdomen)?

Answer The macrocosmic alchemical agent is the union of both outer and inner microcosmic agents which emits the light of Reality. The nectar (or sweet dew, kan lu) is produced long after the intermingling of the four symbols (prenatal heaven and earth and postnatal heart and abdomen) and the union of the sun with the moon (the positive yang and negative yin). He who knows how to gather it will obtain the golden nectar but he who does not gets only the white one (pure saliva). If it is young the light is blurred and unstable in the chung kung cavity (solar plexus). This (circle of) light manifests in the condition of utter stillness but if it grows from a small to a large one and then vanishes, or if it shrinks from a large to a small

one, splits into three, or looks like a crescent, all this shows that
the generative force and vitality are not full. But if the light
suddenly goes up and down so quickly that the eyes cannot
follow it, it is imperative to gather vitality immediately and
return the circle of light to the body. Then after his heart and
intellect have settled the practiser should roll his eyes from A
to D, G, J and back to A, as follows:[2]

$$\begin{array}{c}
\text{G(3)} \\
\text{J(4)} \swarrow \quad \text{Eyes} \quad \nwarrow \text{D(2)} \\
\text{A(1)} \\
\searrow \qquad \nearrow
\end{array}$$

After rolling his eyes, he should close them and as his
mouth is now full of golden nectar, he should make pointed
concentration on the vitality which he has just circulated (as
above), driving it down (the jen mo or channel of function),
followed by the golden nectar, into the cavity of vitality (below
the navel). This is returning vitality to the cauldron to seal it
there.

After the golden nectar has been swallowed with a gulp
that echoes loudly in the belly, the practiser should draw the
pupils of his eyes close to each other (see page 82) to
concentrate on the cavity of vitality (the lower tan t'ien under
the navel) for a long while so that the light which disappeared
at the previous sitting manifests again. This is the method of
gathering prenatal basic vitality.

Chang Tzu Yang said: 'After nature and life have been
returned to the macrocosm there is no reason why the
practiser should fail to produce the golden elixir (chin t'an).'

The patriarch Lu Tsu said: 'The union of nature and life
is the foundation of Tao and the harmony of the five elements

[2]These four cardinal points are in the same order as in the microcosmic orbit.

(of metal, wood, water, fire and earth) produces the elixir of immortality.'

My master Liao K'ung said: 'Nature and life cannot be sublimated in one day; so hurry to gather and keep them in the body.'

My brother Kuei I Tsu said: 'Gather the prenatal vitality that appears (between the eyes) in front of the original cavity of spirit and roll your eyes to drive it into the lower tan t'ien (under the navel).'

Shun I Tsu said: 'Man has two bodies, the physical which is tangible and the spiritual which is intangible. The physical body is that given by our parents, and the spiritual is prenatal vitality produced by the first six methods of practice (Chapters 1 to 6) and is our essential nature. The Mysterious Gate, from the Ultimateless (wu chi) to the Supreme Ultimate (t'ai chi), reveals that circle (of light) which is (the manifestation of the) real nature of the self.'

A student should begin his practice with real nature in order to develop the heavenly (macrocosmic) body so that his true spirit can emerge from his heart. For form relies on spirit to be free from decay, and spirit relies on (essential) nature to be immune from death. So we know that this real nature embodies both (essential) nature and (eternal) life, and is symbolised by a circle which stands for its immaterial substance, free from decay, which is its spiritual body; and that all material forms are subject to destruction.

Therefore, the secret lies in the prenatal positive vitality that existed before heaven, earth and all things came into being; which is perfect, bright, pure and clean; with nothing screening it and immune against all contamination. It is that circle (of light) appearing before the eyes, which is true nature exposed by the sublimation of nature and life.

Question Is this circle one's real face before one was born; (if so) what are its form and shape?

Answer This circle manifests through the faithful cultivation of (essential) nature and (eternal) life. A diligent trainee is bound to realise the light of vitality which is red and reveals the blood-coloured (spurious) Mysterious Gate and when white shows the genuine gate which has neither beginning nor end, is neither changeable nor transformable, neither existing nor non-existent; neither round nor square, neither excessive nor deficient, neither increasing nor decreasing, neither coming nor going, neither created nor destroyed, neither within nor without, neither yellow nor red, neither white nor blue, and neither sound nor smell; seeming to be real yet unreal, and dead yet alive. It functions in activity and is hidden when inactive. There is no fixed time for it to come in and out, and its whereabouts is undiscoverable. Since time immemorial it has existed between heaven and earth, being the core of all things and the root of rebirth and transformation. Heaven, earth and all things owe their existence to it and he who knows this circle can recognise his original face before a body was given him by his parents.

Question Chapter 4 teaches circulating (vitality) through the four cardinal points from A to D, G and J; Chapter 6 teaches the ascent of positive and descent of negative fire and also circulating (vitality) through the four cardinal points A, D, G and J; and Chapter 7 again teaches circulating (vitality) through the four cardinal points A, D, G and J. I am really confused and pray you to enlighten me.

Answer These three methods of turning the eyes round have different purposes: (a) macrocosmic sublimation of the generative force, (b) microcosmic purification of vitality and

(c) gathering vitality to invigorate spirit. All three aim at sublimating the generative force, vitality and spirit.

(a) The macrocosmic sublimation of generative force aims at gathering the alchemical agent during the (various) phases of the circulation of fire (in the microcosmic orbit as explained earlier). In order to gather the alchemical agent the practiser should roll his eyes which stand for the sun and the moon. This is likened to the sun's orbit of 365¼ degrees; hence the macrocosm.

When the generative and vital forces start vibrating the practiser should roll his eyes from A through D to F (see *figure 2* on page 15) to lift positive fire which will cover thirty-six degrees in six phases or 216 degrees, and then from G through J to L to lower its negative counterpart which will embrace twenty-four degrees in six phases or 144 degrees.

Thus each combined ascent and descent of fire embraces 360 degrees with pauses for cleansing and purifying at D and J. The difference of five and a quarter degrees spreads between the four cardinal points A, D, G and J for the microcosmic orbiting with temporary pauses whereas the sun and the moon continue to orbit endlessly in heaven.

The rolling of the eyes to gather the alchemical agent and the rise of the gentle breeze (regulated breathing) show that both spirit and vitality move together.

The Tan Ching says: 'Spirit is aroused by rolling the eyes and vitality by breathing which sets the generative and vital forces in motion.'

This is macrocosmic sublimation of the generative force but if cleansing and purifying are omitted the generative and vital forces mingle with each other and cannot be separated (for alchemical purposes).

(b) The microcosmic sublimation of vitality has been

taught in Chapter 6. The method consists of rolling the eyes nine times in each of the four phases (from A to D, G and J) or thirty-six times in all to raise positive fire for the purpose of shutting the Mysterious Gate (pi kuan), and then of rolling the eyes six times in each of the four phases (from G to D, A and J) or twenty-four times in all to lower negative fire for the purpose of opening the Mysterious Gate (k'ai kuan). These turns pass through the four cardinal points A, D, G and J for the purpose of sublimating the generative force already gathered into vitality. But if cleansing and purifying are omitted the generative force cannot be entirely transmuted into vitality.

(c) This chapter teaches the method of gathering prenatal basic vitality in order to invigorate spirit thereby linking the four positive and negative principles (szu ko yin yang) (see page 77) to produce the macrocosmic alchemical agent. When the light of vitality manifests it reveals the formation of that agent; and its subtle functioning discloses (the presence of) spirit.

The practiser should hold spirit and vitality together in front of the original cavity of spirit (tsu ch'iao between and behind the eyes) so that all three (the generative force, vitality and spirit) unite into one whole. To achieve this, he should first freeze spirit to return it to primeval darkness until in this condition of utter stillness it radiates and illumines the whole of empty space; and then hold on to the centre (between and behind the eyes) to realise the oneness for the purpose of returning to the source.

While the centre is being held on to to realise this oneness, the light of spirit is still young and unstable and if it tends to run away or change, the practiser should roll his eyes from A to D, G and J and back to A (i.e. through the four cardinal points of the microcosmic orbit) concentrating on driving vitality back into the lower tan t'ien cavity (under the navel). When vitality returns to its source life is boundless. This is the transmutation of basic vitality to invigorate spirit which is 'my' spirit of no spirit (i.e. the inexpressible).

Hence my master Liao K'ung said: 'As the dragon and tiger "copulate" and the sun and the moon unite, a mysterious pearl will be created in the middle of the state of indistinctness.'

My eldest brother K'uei I Tsu said: 'When positive and negative (principles) unite to return to the centre (of the Mysterious Gate), if vitality is young and tends to scatter, you should rotate the solar disc (to check it).' (See *figure* 5 on page 72)

This is what the Chin Hsien Cheng Lun says when dealing with 'risk full of perils': 'If the practiser does not continue with right concentration he will miss the chance to achieve (the above) "copulation and union".' It adds: 'If the mind is truly set on gathering and union, basic vitality will be stable and will not scatter; it will then help the alchemical pregnancy which is the outcome of cultivating both (essential) nature and (eternal) life.'

This seventh step is referred to in the Hsin Yin Ching which says: 'The method of using the three components of the alchemical agent (the generative force, vitality and spirit) consists of driving the first two into the third to invigorate it.'

Hence Liu Hua Yang said: 'A long practice will mature the generative force to transmute it into vitality, for the generative force is only immature vitality.' He also said: 'The generative force and vitality are inseparable. Only a good understanding of the union of sun and moon can lead to real achievement.'

Question You have said that the first six steps (Chapters 1 to 6) contribute to the full development of positive spirit as revealed by the light of vitality which is called the Mysterious Gate, positive spirit or original face. In spite of its many names it is only the radiant circle or ball of light (mentioned earlier). Although I have only recently begun to practise, I realise this bright white light after the first step; is it the true nature as revealed by the Mysterious Gate?

Answer You have only realised the negative spirit which appears during the preliminary step of practice. When you close your eyes and see a white light in front of you it is negative spirit which is absolutely useless. By practising all the first six steps you will gather the outer and inner alchemical agent and so restore the generative force to invigorate the brain so that the positive spirit manifests. The light of vitality thus seen while your eyes are open is the Mysterious Gate which reveals the real nature realised by cultivating both (essential) nature and (eternal) life, which is the secret of alchemy.

If you wrongly search for negative spirit by closing your eyes to look into the (relative) emptiness of the void it will lead to (the realm of) birth and death, which is in the province of consciousness; you will then achieve nothing until you die. But if you follow the first six steps to gather the alchemical agent according to the doctrine of the cultivation of both (essential) nature and (eternal) life, you will realise the positive spirit which is the outcome of meditation on the void that is not empty (i.e. is the absolute) and is beyond birth and death. The spirit thus created is beyond spirit itself for the light of (essential) nature comes from the ultimateless (wu chi) which manifests when your body is full of prenatal generative force and disappears when the latter is lacking. The presence of this light of (essential) nature leads to life whereas its absence causes death. The cultivation of both nature and life leads to the realisation of this light of prenatal vitality whereas the production of postnatal negative spirit results in con-sciousness.

8

PLUNGING SPIRIT INTO THE LOWER TAN T'IEN CAVITY

This method consists of driving into the cavity of vitality (below the navel) the positive spirit which has gathered in front of its original cavity (tsu ch'iao between and behind the eyes) and is called plunging spirit into the lower tan t'ien centre. This centre (under the navel) has outer and inner cells; the outer cell is the source of the positive and negative principles, which is the abode of (vital) breath, the spring of foetal breathing and the mechanism of in and out breathing; the inner is where the Tao foetus is created and the (vital) breath stays, and is the home of serenity. When the (inner) vital breath moving up and down in the body, does not go up beyond the heart or down beyond the lower abdomen, it becomes the real (or stabilised vital) breath which will in time enter this cavity (under the navel to stay there) causing the sudden manifestation of true serenity.

The purpose of the previous seventh step (Chapter 7) in the practice of alchemy is like providing a barren woman with all that she needs to make her capable of bearing children. The true seed (foetus) thus realised comes from the habitual restraint of anger and passion, silent meditation and quieting of mind which lead to the destruction of the mortal heart (mind) and the resurrection of Tao (immortal) heart (mind). For the death of the earthly heart exposes the moonlight of (essential) nature which is always screened by the dust of passions so long as the mortal mind is allowed to exist.

The student, awakened to the teaching, should strive to control his heart (the house of fire) by driving his mind into the field of concentration so as to still and disengage it from sense data. When the mind stops wandering outside, consciousness will melt away, and the five aggregates will be empty of externals so that spirit and vitality will gather and stay within and no longer scatter without.

The body is the abode of (vital) breath and the heart (the house of fire) is the temple of spirit. If vitality is cut off spirit will lose support and cannot stay in the heart for an instant. Therefore, a practiser enjoying good health will feel his vital breath vibrate in his body after practising meditation for a long time, and he will finally perceive his original face which is the light of (essential) nature. He will feel unusual comfort, and by concentrating on spirit to gather vitality he will thereby cultivate (eternal) life; only then can the goal of cultivating (eternal) life be attained.

He should wait until the light becomes red and vibrates to gather immediately prenatal vitality which is bound to disperse if it is not kept in cold storage in the lower tan t'ien cavity (under the navel).

This method of cold storage consists of driving the light of prenatal positive spirit from its original cavity (tsu ch'iao between and behind the eyes) down into the lower abdomen with a loud noise which confirms that the bottom of that centre is reached. The practiser should then turn inwards his eyes to concentrate on the lower tan t'ien as long as possible until its inner heat vibrates. He should then imagine that this vitality is lifted to the heart (the house of fire) and lowered to the lower abdomen (the house of water), with continued ascents and descents (in the ch'ung mo or thrusting channel) until all of a sudden it slips into the cavity of vitality (under the navel); this is called 'entry into the cavity within a cavity' and is actual 're-entry into the foetus for further creativity' which is the outcome of linking the heart with the abdomen.

When a man sleeps soundly, the element of fire in spirit goes down to scorch the element of water in the lower abdomen which will be transformed into steam that will soar up linking the heart and lower abdomen. When he wakes up and opens his eyes, spirit returns to his organ of sight thereby disengaging the heart from the lower abdomen which will not reunite even if he starves for a week. Why? Because of the exhaustion of prenatal vitality whose source of supply has been cut off. This man will thus lose the means to preserve life.

Question I am stupid and do not understand the method of freezing spirit in the cavity of vitality (under the navel). Will you please explain in detail?

Answer It is the consolidating method which consists of turning back the seeing and hearing *to* empty the heart (of sense data) so as to freeze spirit and so gather vitality which will then stop draining away. Only by daily practice of holding on to the centre of vitality (under the navel) to realise the oneness (of all things) can the union of heart and lower abdomen be achieved in the state of (mental) stillness. This can never be done by worldly men in their sleep.

Now let us examine the human body. The usual drain of vitality through the heavenly pool (tien chih) cavity in the mouth can be stopped by raising the tongue to touch the palate (in order to make a bridge so that vitality can flow into the throat and chest before returning (in the jen mo channel) to its centre below the navel). But far more of it drains through the genital gate than through the heavenly pool and if this is not checked it can kill even chaste youths.

Therefore, the vitality normally lost in this way should be made good by alchemical means in order to return it to its source to restore (eternal) life and so preserve the body. Hence 'boundless life' but if vitality is not preserved and the discharge of generative force continues the practiser will remain mortal like all worldlings, for if spirit wanders outside, vitality will scatter to become generative fluid the exhaustion of which leads to death.

Man lives and dies because of his body. This body comes into being because of the pregnancy of a woman due to the union of her generative force with that of a man through the mortal gate in their bodies. Before the umbilical cord is cut, the (baby's essential) nature and (eternal) life are inseparable: this state is called prenatal. This body is mortal because of the postnatal condition of nature and life which are no longer united but divided into two, and so become unconnected.

When the child grows up he searches for the opposite sex and gives rise to sexual desires and so exhausts whatever remains of his prenatal positive principle in its *positive* condition. Henceforth he must rely on food and drink to obtain the positive principle in its *negative* state to make good the deficiency. Since he does not realise the importance of nature and life, he indulges in all kinds of excesses and that positive principle in its negative state becomes inadequate to sustain his life. How then can he escape from death?

Therefore, we should know that the birth of a body is followed by its death. Now in order to avoid mortality, the self-natured spirit should re-enter the foetus anew in order to produce (essential) nature and (eternal) life once more.

The method consists at the start of collecting spirit to drive it into the cavity of vitality (under the navel) so that vitality will envelop spirit until when utter stillness prevails both will gather and unite into a whole which will slip into that cavity where it will remain in an unperturbed state called the immortal (Tao) foetus. This foetus is not a real one having form and shape; for it is an incorporeal manifestation of the union of spirit with vitality. It is unlike an ordinary foetus, the outcome of desire and love. He who wants his body of flesh and blood to become immortal is like someone rubbing a brick to make a bright mirror, which is impossible.

Question Taoist teaching seems to lay more stress on the cultivation of (eternal) life while neglecting that of (essential) nature. Only Chapter 1 deals with '*fixing spirit in its original cavity* (between and behind the eyes)' which pertains to nature. Why does the teaching deal more with life than nature?

Answer Chapter 1 deals with '*fixing spirit in its original cavity*', for man's body, spirit, intellect, incorporeal (hun) and corporeal (p'o) souls are all negative (yin) and obey the heart's impulses. When the heart is still so are all these five, but when it moves they all move as well. Self-realisation consists of transmuting this human heart into an immortal one; hence the saying: 'the cultivation of heart to preserve (essential) nature'. The profound method of preserving nature does not go beyond the paths of the tu mo (controlling) and jen mo (functioning) channels.

In your daily meditation if you cannot set your heart at rest in order to fix spirit in its original cavity (in the centre of the brain between and behind the eyes), you should rely on the working of the stove and cauldron and on the channels of control and function so that you can stop the thinking process.

If you succeed in holding on to that cavity you will immediately realise the state of serenity; but if you fail, this is due solely to your remissness.

All eight (psychic) channels are clear in the prenatal state but prenatal vitality is cut off after a man falls into postnatal condition (i.e. when the umbilical cord has been cut). Therefore, it is important to study Chapter 3 and practise its teaching in order to keep all psychic channels clear so that vitality and blood circulate freely in the body and thereby wipe out all ailments.

If you do not practise meditation you will never achieve this wonderful result. When the genital organ is aroused and stands erect during your meditation, you should practise the method taught in Chapter 4 and when you are familiar with the inner mechanism, you will be able to transmute the generative force into vitality.

If after sitting for a long time you still fail to experience the arousal of the genital organ, there must be something wrong in the viscera. Then read Chapter 5 and practise its teaching to get rid of all inner causes of ailments.

When the positive principle manifests thereby transmuting the generative force into vitality, if you do not know the teaching in Chapter 6 and cannot avoid the risks involved, vitality will turn into generative force. In that case you should practise the ascent of positive and descent of negative fire in order to transmute vitality into spirit until the light of (essential) nature manifests in front of you; only then can you lay the foundation of immortality. However, if stirrings and thoughts continue to arise and if your heart (the house of fire) is not settled, spirit will wander outside and (vital) breath will disperse; the foundation thus laid will be destroyed.

Therefore, it is most important that you lay down all thoughts in order to restore the foundation you have achieved, and read Chapter 7 which teaches the return of spirit to nothingness; only then can you avoid the risk of spirit returning to the state of vitality.

Both this chapter and the previous one are very closely related and the student who has successfully practised the teachings in both will enter the immortal path.

Immortality is attained after the successful cultivation of (essential) nature; this is why in Chapter 1 we began by teaching concentration on the original cavity of spirit (tsu ch'iao between and behind the eyes). For he who succeeds in cultivating nature, can expect to realise (eternal) life as well.

Question What do you mean by the union of the male element of metal with the female element of wood?

Answer The male element of metal is the sun and the female element of wood is the moon. After a man has fallen into the postnatal state (i.e. has been born), he loses the power of concentration; this is why his sun and moon do not unite. If he understands the profound meaning of their union and concentrates on the cavity of the dragon (lung kung below the navel) until they both unite, true vitality will manifest of itself.

The cavity of the dragon is (the lower tan t'ien under the navel) which is the seat of the element of water and contains the original vital force. The heart is the seat of the element of fire and contains the original spirit. The method consists of concentrating on the lower abdomen under the navel thereby directing the element of fire in spirit down to the northern sea (the lower tan t'ien) wherein the element of water, being scorched, will evaporate and become steam that soars up.

The immersion of fire in water causes their 'copulation' and the resultant condition is called '*fire and water in stable equilibrium*' (shui huo chi chi). If the outer sun and moon do not mingle their lights the inner water and fire do not 'copulate' and prenatal true vitality cannot manifest. If they are left to themselves to follow their postnatal course the element of fire will remain dry and that of water will continue wet, with the former soaring up and the latter going down, both running in opposite directions. If water is not scorched by fire it will not evaporate to become steam that soars up. This is the unstable state of water and fire as shown by the story of the cowherd and weaving maiden in the Nei Ching.[1]

Fire is hot and soars up; it is symbolised by the maiden who weaves hard day and night, is likened to the heart (the seat of fire) which is impermanent, refuses to relinquish worldly attachments and is subject to the endless round of birth and death. Water is wet and flows down; it is symbolised by the cowherd tilling the soil without respite, who stands for vitality that scatters easily; when the latter is exhausted he will have no time even to turn his head (to think of himself).

Taoist alchemy uses the (planetary) signs in heaven to teach the method of preparing the elixir of immortality with analogies which are very profound and are not meant to deceive (and harm) others.

Hsu Ching Yang said: 'If the macrocosmic elixir of immortality is not produced by intermingling the lights of the sun and moon, and the union of heaven with earth, what can make it?' This is the wonderful union of the elements of metal and wood.

---

[1]According to Chinese mythology, to the east of the heavenly river lived a maiden who worked hard to weave heavenly robes. The heavenly king took pity on her loneliness and allowed her to marry a cowherd living to the west of the river. After being married, she stopped working and the king was angry and ordered her to return to the east, permitting her to cross the river to meet her husband only once a year on the seventh day of the seventh month.

This story shows the unstable states of the female element of water and the male element of fire which cause hurnan sufferings.

Question Will you please enlighten me on the various stages of sublimation during the microcosmic orbiting?

Answer The microcosmic orbit is also called the wheel of the law. Wind and fire are used to drive vitality through the (psychic) channels of control (tu mo in the spine) and of function (jen mo in the front of the body). When starting the exercise, inhalation and exhalation should succeed each other to stop all external disturbances so that spirit and vitality can unite. The practiser will feel warmth below the navel, and this feeling may later last for the whole day. He will then notice that positive vitality will first rise from the base of the spine; it will in time, as his practice continues, go up the backbone, and if his determination is firm, will pierce through the occiput to reach the top of his head. So if he has been taught the secret of alchemy, he can drive this positive vitality through the three gates (in the channel of control) at once.

For when positive vitality manifests it always tends to sink and disperse. Spirit can hold vitality only temporarily but lacks the driving power of breathing, and without breathing, vitality cannot be driven into the channels of control and function (to circulate in the microcosmic orbit) and will finally drain away by the genital gate; this is caused by the lack of pressure from in and out breathing.

When practising alchemy, the student should shut his mouth and roll up his tongue (to make a bridge as explained earlier). When he inhales postnatal (fresh) air should enter by the nostrils and the throat gradually reaching the lower tan t'ien cavity (under the navel) simultaneously he should lift his concentration from the mortal cavity (at the root of the penis) up the spine until it reaches the top of his head. When he exhales postnatal air should go out through the throat and nostrils; simultaneously he should drop his concentration from the top of the head (in the channel of function) to the spot between the eyebrows (in front of the cavity of spirit), behind the tongue, and down the throat to the chiang kung cavity (in the solar plexus) and the centre of vitality (below the navel) until he reaches the gate of mortality (at the root of the penis) where he should stop. This circulation should go on endlessly until the two cavities of (essential) nature (in the heart) and (eternal) life (under the navel) vibrate, heralding the production of true vitality.

If the practiser looks back he will remember that his practices seemed to be aimless turnings of the wheel of the law. For if he fails to catch positive vitality it cannot be produced, and even if it could be it would finally disperse through other channels in the body. When, however, the wheel of the law stops of itself and is followed by a state of serenity, it should be let alone and not forced to turn. Vitality may then soar up or the penis may stand erect. In this case the microcosmic orbiting should be stopped so that 'the flute without holes' can be played to check if vitality is genuine or not. If the latter is spurious the penis will shrink but if it is genuine it will remain erect.

The patriarch Liu Hua Yang said: 'No Taoist function is better than the wheel of the law and no line of communication is better than the immortal path. The wheel of the law is true vitality and the path is the (orbit through the) channels of control (tu mo) and function (jen mo). All those who followed my words have now reached their goals.'

For the benefit of readers I now repeat the instructions given me by my masters.

My elder brother K'uei I Tsu said: 'When the sun and the moon *without* unite (i.e. when the pupils of both eyes are drawn close to each other in a squint for pointed concentration), the heart (the house of fire) and lower abdomen (the house of water) *within* are automatically linked; only then can prenatal vitality develop gradually. When the (functionings of the) heart and lower abdomen are inverted, that is when the former is lowered and the latter lifted, serenity will in time be achieved. When advancing further in the training, if the practiser, instead of cultivating (eternal) life, merely closes his eyes to freeze his heart and so disengages all six sense organs, thereby cutting all links between the front and back as well as the upper and lower parts of the body, how can he develop prenatal vitality? Students should pay attention to all this.

The Wu Chen P'ien says:

> Before the elixir is produced move not to the mountain
> Where lead (vitality) is found neither within nor without.
> This gem is self-possessed in every man
> Who usually ignores its existence.

This means that the precious gem is inherent in every man's body and that achievement does not depend solely on stillness in the mountain.

My old master Liao K'ung said: 'Even if you are still not clear about heaven and earth, the sun and moon, the heart (house of fire) and lower abdomen (house of water) and the centre (of the four cardinal points) (see *figure 4* on page 35) you can gather the light as expounded in Chapter 7 and drive it into your lower abdomen by concentrating on the lower tan t'ien cavity there, until true vitality in time vibrates and rises to the chiang kung centre (in the solar plexus) where it will stay for a little before returning to the lower tan t'ien where it will vibrate there for some time before returning to stillness. Suddenly it will re-enter the cavity of vitality (below the navel) where it will stay still; this is the state of utter serenity (ta ting) which reveals the linking of heart and lower abdomen, and the centralisation of all four cardinal points, also called 'the stable equilibrium of water and fire (shui huo chi chi).'

The return of vitality to the lower tan t'ien (under the navel) after spirit has been fixed in its original cavity (in the centre of the brain between and behind the eyes, see Chapter 1) will, after one day and night of stillness, enable the practiser to abstain from food for a week; and by advancing further he will be able to stop eating for seven weeks. Only then can he dwell in real serenity.

The old master T'an Chih Ming said: 'After gathering the alchemical agent to make good the loss of generative force, a fascinating white light will appear in both eyes' which means the joining up of the sun (the left eye or the male principle) with the moon (the right eye or female principle); only then can both eyes be concentrated on the lower abdomen in which a white light is imagined as manifesting. After looking into the lower tan t'ien for several tens of days suddenly a sound will be heard, followed by the ascent of real vitality from the lower belly to the heart (the house of fire) where it stays still, thence going down to return to the lower tan t'ien. This daily exercise without counting the number of days, will decrease the number of in and out breaths and strip the heart (the seat of fire) of thoughts and stirrings while no trace of the body can be found; this is the state of deep serenity.

9

THE IMMORTAL BREATHING OR THE SELF-WINDING WHEEL OF THE LAW

The shutting (ho) and opening (p'i) process of immortal breathing causes postnatal vital breath to rise from the heels up to the channel of control through which it soars to the brain, thence going down in the channel of function to the trunk (i.e. the mortal gate). These continual ascents and descents will in time vibrate prenatal true vitality in the lower tan t'ien which will first ascend in the channel of control to the brain to push postnatal vital breath there down in the channel of function to the trunk, and will then descend in the channel of function to the base of the penis to drive postnatal vital breath up in the channel of control to the brain.

In the last chapter we explained the method of freezing spirit which is so called because it consists of first gathering prenatal true vitality in the original cavity of spirit (tsu ch'iao in the centre of the brain) and then driving it into the lower tan t'ien (under the navel). When doing it the eyes should turn inward to look into the latter centre until the heart and intellect are disengaged from the duality of the self and others and unite in the state of indistinctness until exhalation becomes subtle while inhalation continues unbroken, harmonic and restful. In time

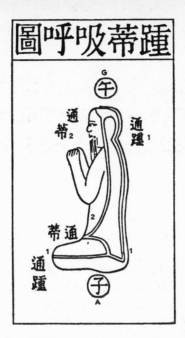

Figure 7 The heel and trunk channels. 1 the heel channel (tung chung) from the heels to the brain. 2 the trunk channel (tung ti) from the lower abdomen to the brain.

the lower tan t'ien centre (under the navel) vibrates extending its field of activity from the heart to the lower belly. After a long time this vibration will stop and be replaced by stillness, with the result that all inner (vital) breaths stop leaving the body whereas all outer ones continue to enter it; this reveals the restoration of foetal breath (see below) and the return (of pre-natal vitality) to its source which is 'a cavity within a cavity'; thus the state of profound serenity is attained.

This profound foetal breathing, now fully restored, neither gathers nor scatters and is disconnected from (the duality of) the self and others; its serenity is lasting, being neither within nor without, neither stillness nor disturbance, and free from vibration; thus it unites the sun with the moon, and joins up the positive and negative principles. It puts an end to the state of confusion and causes the practiser to enter the (immortal) foetus to clear away all postnatal conditions.

This foetal breathing depends neither on breathing through the nostrils or mouth nor on retaining the breath in the lower tan t'ien. Outsiders and heretics use the nostrils or mouth to breathe only fresh air, a process which bears no relation to the production of the elixir of immortality in the cultivation of both (essential) nature and (eternal) life.

Postnatal vital breath is 'inhaled' through the heels and 'exhaled' through the trunk for the purpose of vibrating prenatal true vitality in the lower tan t'ien (under the navel). So an in-breath from the heels to lift postnatal breath in the channel of control is followed by an out-breath from the trunk to lower it in the channel of function, and, as time passes, these continued ascents and descents will set in motion prenatal true vitality in the lower tan t'ien centre, which will then automatically rise in the channel of control to the brain causing postnatal vital breath there to sink in the channel of function to the mortal gate. When prenatal true vitality drops in the channel of function to the mortal gate, it forces postnatal vital breath there to go up in the channel of control to the brain. These are four movements of postnatal vital breath and prenatal true vitality without the breathing of outer air through the nostrils or mouth coming into play. If these ascents and descents are caused by air breathed in and out by the nostrils or mouth they have nothing to do with the immortal breathing which operates of itself independently of the practiser's will.

The circulation of prenatal vitality is to produce the bright pearl, and the method consists of using postnatal (vital) breath to blow and stir the lower tan t'ien cavity (under the navel) where both prenatal vitality and postnatal vital breath drive each other up and down as already described.

When so regulating the postnatal (vital) breath the practiser should concentrate on the cavity of vitality (the lower tan t'ien under the navel) in order to transmute prenatal vitality into a bright pearl. Walking, standing, rising and reclining (in the performance of daily work) are all appropriate times for turning the wheel of the law, the purpose of which is to sublimate prenatal vitality in order to nurture eternal life. This prenatal vitality should move in unison with postnatal (vital) breath in unbroken continuity; this is the self-winding wheel of the law which is the macrocosm.

When the practiser reaches this stage, he should guard against any drain of the positive principle at night, for if he is careless the original generative force will disperse and thereby nullify all that has been achieved. I urge all serious students to pay particular attention to this.

If his effort slackens for a single day he will be disturbed by dreams at night and will thereby lose the prenatal generative force. He should know that all diligent practisers are free from dreams. The Tan Ching says: 'The perfect man is free from dreams.' This does not mean that he does not have dreams but he is free from bad ones. There are four categories of good men who are free from bad dreams: the perfect, the immortal, the saint and the sage.[1]

Lustful and gluttonous worldly men can still practise (alchemy) which is really difficult for drowsy people. When a worldly man sees something attractive in his dream others near

[1]Chih jen, the perfect man in whom moral virtues and learned accomplishments reach the highest point; chen jen, the immortal who is no longer ruled by what he sees, hears and feels; sheng jen, the saintly man who is divinely inspired and intuitively wise; and hsien jen, the sage, a man of excellent virtues.

him see nothing. In his dream he may walk the streets, pick a beautiful flower, hear someone speak to him, make or lose money, and all these things are unreal. But when he dreams of involuntary emission he really experiences a discharge of generative fluid. Therefore, all dreams are unreal except that of emission which is followed by the discharge of the generative fluid.

If the practiser wants to overcome drowsiness in order to be free from dreams, he should use the method called *'coiling up the body into five dragons'* which will stop his drowsiness and put an end to his dreams; as a result his nocturnal emissions will stop and he will no longer have to worry about the loss of this most precious thing that preserves life. He will then be able to sublimate generative force into the bright pearl.

To achieve this he should rely on the fourfold alchemical process of breathing: *inhalation, exhalation, ascent* and *descent* which produce the immortal breath which is independent of breathing through the nostrils or mouth.

The patriarch Wu Ch'ung Hsu said:
Who says that sublimation by fire cannot be taught
Since only silent circuits can plumb the depth sublime?
In days of old thousands of saintly men realised this by
looking
Clearly into their breathing process to win immortality

By stoppage of respiration is meant the condition of serenity in which the practiser becomes unconscious, his breathing (almost) ceases and his pulses (all but) stop beating. This is called freezing spirit.

The first eight chapters of this book deal with the condition of minor serenity (hsiao ting ching) and the present chapter with the stoppage of (ordinary) breathing which implies major serenity (ta ting ching).

When the practiser first achieves the state of stillness he realises only minor serenity which lasts one day in which dullness and confusion cause him to be unconscious, like a dying man who is breathless. Then he will experience medium serenity lasting three successive days, and major serenity lasting seven successive days. This third stage should not be mistaken for death (by transformation) for it only reveals the return of spirit and vitality to the source, the revival of (eternal) life and the sublimation of the alchemical agent into a bright pearl.

The practiser now needs good care from his companions who should avoid disturbing his positive spirit in its serenity. On no account should he avail himself on this revival of (eternal) life to come out of the state of serenity. He should see to it that because of this still vitality his spirit will enter by itself the major serenity in which his prenatal immaculate vitality will spring from nothingness.

An ancient immortal said: 'Men are subject to birth and death because they breathe in and out by the nostrils and mouth; if they (practically) cease breathing they will realise immortality.' For if the practiser (almost) ceases to breathe he will achieve major serenity. When the breath remains (nearly) stationary, the (immortal) foetus will be as secure as a mountain and by continuing his practice he will achieve minor and major serenity; all phenomena will be absorbed into nothingness and with spirit frozen in this state by day and night, the bright pearl will form in this unperturbed nothingness. If this serenity is not achieved the immortal seed cannot be produced. The moment when he enters this serenity is likened to his approaching death that precedes the resurrection which is the main object of alchemy. As to how death is followed by resurrection, this concerns the method of producing the bright pearl.

When (essential) nature and (eternal) life unite in the confused state in the cavity of vitality (under the navel) the least carelessness on the part of the practiser may cause his failure to keep them together there; spirit will then leave this centre and the most precious thing will drain away at night. This is the most critical moment when he will either preserve or injure (eternal) life. And so he should be determined firmly to preserve this serenity at all costs by concentrating his spirit pointedly on this cavity, which is the most important thing at this stage of training.

An ancient immortal said: 'The first stirring thought threw me into the sea of suffering; now the first subsiding thought (saves me by) sending me to the other shore (of liberation) for a single (stirring) thought causes the round of birth and death.'

If the practiser feels that his body is cold and breathes out cold air this is due to wrong practice without prior instruction from competent masters. This negative state comes from an interruption of the inner (vital) breath which stops giving support to spirit fixed in the cavity of vitality (below the navel) thereby cooling the inner fire in the lower tan t'ien and preventing the light of the elixir from manifesting. This negative state is also due to many other causes but the chief one is the cooling of the lower tan t'ien centre.

The Fa Chueh says: 'To remedy this negative state requires concentration of true inner fire which is done by fixing spirit in the lower tan t'ien, the source of foetal breath, by drawing the pupils of the eyes close to each other in order to bring the cavity of vitality into focus and by using the bellows to bring quick fire into action; as a result of pointed concentration a mass of true inner fire will soar up causing spiritual light in the cauldron to illuminate the whole body the four elements of which (see note 3 on page 47) are thereby sublimated. It will eliminate this malefic negative state and restore the brightness of the elixir in its cavity (under the navel).'

This cultivation of (essential) nature and (eternal) life requires constant attention and the slightest carelessness can obscure the inner light and cause the drain of the elixir with the result that all previous efforts will be sterile.

There are also meditators who (inadvertently) arouse the evil fire in the liver and kidneys which blurs their vision, and causes them to see double, their eyes to become astigmatic, the pupils to enlarge and the white to redden.

If the practiser wants to avoid stirring this evil fire which can drain away the 'precious thing' at night, he should know that the trouble is caused by unwholesome food and intoxicating drink, by perverse thoughts and desires, by hot baths which scatter the heat of the elixir and by (uncontrolled) fire that scorches the body. This has many causes but mainly results from not taking precautions against the misuse of fire during the training. The practiser may also feel hot in the heart which causes him to be parched with thirst and to eat and drink too much. If he fails to overcome this fire his 'most precious thing' will drain away at night.

The practiser should know how to remedy this defect. If it derives from fire in the liver and kidneys, he should practise the method taught in Chapter 5 to eliminate it. If it comes from fire in the heart or from unwholesome food and drink, he should, while sitting in meditation, imagine in front of him a black ball or a dark cloud the size of a fist which he should gather as taught in Chapter 7; he should make pointed concentration to take hold of the black object firmly, breathe in fresh air to drive it into the lower tan t'ien (under the navel) and breathe out slowly to expel the inner evil fire which will then vanish; he will then feel truly at ease.

There is no fixed number of inhalations to drive the dark object into the lower abdomen and of exhalations to expel the malefic fire, but they should be continued until the evil fire is completely extinguished. Henceforth the practiser will enjoy great comfort with enduring high spirits and no more drain of vitality.

Question You have spoken of the fourfold immortal breathing which is not through the nostrils and mouth but alchemical; if so through which channels should it enter and leave the body?

Answer If postnatal (vital) breath is harnessed to vibrations in the lower tan t'ien centre (under the navel) prenatal vitality will ascend while postnatal (vital) breath will descend, and vice versa; these alternating ascents and descents which make four movements up and down are not caused by breathing through the nostrils and mouth, but by postnatal inner breath which starts from the heels and the mortal gate (at the root of the penis); this is postnatal (vital) breath which while descending and ascending drives prenatal vitality up the channel of control (tu mo in the spine) to the brain and thence down through the channel of function (jen mo) to the cavity of mortality, that is ascent and descent of prenatal vitality in these two main channels.

Therefore, these four movements of prenatal vitality and postnatal (vital) breath are independent of breathing through the nostrils and mouth. If postnatal (vital) breath is not properly channelled in its ascent from the heels to the head and its descent thence to the mortal gate, it is far better not to practise this method. For if the nostrils and mouth are used to breathe air in and out at random in the practice of alchemy at this advanced stage, prenatal vitality will burst the psychic centre in the heart with the result that the practiser will become deranged, singing and dancing foolishly, talking nonsense, reciting strange poems, speaking of obscure things, and boasting that he has achieved supreme truth, without realising that all this comes from consciousness which stirs his heart (the house of fire) and dislodges his spirit from its original cavity (in the centre of the brain), thereby shaking his brain and nervous system and causing mental disorders; as a result he will cry or laugh, and feel sad or happy for no apparent cause. This is due to the vitality in the heart which stirs his spirit and makes him so restless that he is unfit for spiritual training. All this is caused by the wrong use of in and out breathing through the nostrils and mouth (in the practice of alchemy at this advanced stage).

In this event the practiser should seek instruction from competent masters who will explain to him that immortal breathing starts from the heels and the mortal gate without passing through the nostrils and mouth. After receiving instruction he should practise the fourfold movement of immortal breathing.

This macrocosmic technique should be practised at all times and in unbroken continuity. It is not true that it cannot be taught to others but it is true that it involves great risks for unguided people.

By way of illustration, when my immortal inhalation reaches my two heels it has actually gone from the original cavity of spirit (tsu ch'iao between and behind the eyes) to the medulla oblongata[2] which is linked with the two psychic channels starting from the heels. As I inhale in this way my concentration also moves from that cavity to the medulla oblongata, pushing up postnatal (vital) breath from the heels

[2]The widening top of the spinal cord which forms the lowest part of the brain and controls breathing, circulation, etc.

into the heel pathway (tung chung) to the base of the spine, thence up the backbone to the back of the head before reaching the brain (ni wan). This shows the heels as the root of immortal inspiration.

When my immortal exhalation returns from the medulla oblongata to the original cavity of spirit (between and behind the eyes) which is linked with the mortal cavity (at the base of the penis) my concentration also moves from the medulla oblongata up to the cavity of spirit driving postnatal (vital) breath (which has reached the brain) into the trunk pathway (tung ti) to the original cavity of spirit, thence down (the jen mo channel) through the throat (and chest to the), chiang kung cavity (the solar plexus) and the lower tan t'ien centre before reaching the mortal gate. This shows that the mortal cavity is the root or immortal exhalation.

Postnatal (vital) breath will thus go up and down independently of ordinary breathing through the nostrils or mouth, and its constant ascent and descent will in time set prenatal vitality in motion so that when the former goes up the latter goes down and vice versa, which is macrocosmic functioning that will continue endlessly without a pause.

My master said: 'When you are perfectly clear about this immortal breathing you will achieve immortality.'

Question You have said that lustful and gluttonous people can practise alchemy, that drowsy people are not fit to practise it and that the perfect man is free from dreams. What is the method of 'coiling up the body into five dragons' which can stop all dreams as well as nocturnal emission?

Answer Lust can be overcome during the six phases of alchemical sublimation which causes the genital organ to retract. Gluttony can be overcome by a vegetarian diet but the practiser should abstain from the five pungent roots (i.e. garlic, three kinds of onions and leeks) which are aphrodisiac and increase the production of generative fluid. But drowsiness is very difficult to overcome; hence the ancients devised a method of sitting continuously in meditation to stop sleeping. Worldly men in their dreams acquire or lose many things such as money or objects and when they wake up they find that it was all unreal; but when they dream of nocturnal emission it is always real. Since the loss of generative fluid is harmful, why do they not call on competent masters for instruction in order to cultivate (essential) nature and (eternal) life?

I have seen corrupt officials who after holding power and amassing a great fortune, could not carry anything away when they died; thus fame and wealth are like things seen in dreams.

But why does nocturnal emission occur (even) when there is no dream? When a man is awake, his consciousness is seated in his eyes, but when he sleeps at night, it is lodged in the lower abdomen. So when he sleeps his breathing disturbs all six senses and arouses the generative force which will drain away; hence his involuntary emission.

To prevent this loss of generative fluid the practiser should, while in bed at night, touch the palate with the tip of the tongue and drive spirit into the lower tan t'ien cavity (under the navel) in order to empty the heart (the house of fire) of all thoughts; he should then breathe in outer air which (in its vital form) will reach the lower tan t'ien where it will unite with vitality. This union of the elements of water (in the lower belly) and of fire (driven from its seat in the heart) will result in subtle, long breaths causing spirit to embrace vitality and vice versa. The practiser will enjoy a sleep which seems to be, yet is not really, deep, that is an automatic repose in which state how can there be nocturnal emission?

There is another method called 'coiling up the body into

116   Taoist Yoga

five dragons' which consists of 'composing' one's head (i.e. putting it in a comfortable position); curving and reclining the body on either side, like the coiled length of a sleeping dragon or the curved body of a dog, bending one arm for a pillow while stretching the other to place a hand on the belly, and straightening one leg while bending the other. Even before the heart is immersed in sleep, the pupils of both eyes should be drawn close to each other for pointed concentration on the great emptiness so that in the condition of utter stillness the vital principle returns automatically to its source (under the navel), breathing continues normally and so is self-regulated, and the (vital) breath is brought under perfect control. This method of sleeping will banish all dreams and so prevent the generative fluid from draining away.

In case of random drowsiness without (first) cutting out impure breaths and stirring thoughts when one falls into deep sleep, the positive breath in the body will be completely submerged by its negative counterpart so that he will be like a dead man. This is because he does not know how to regulate his breathing.

Question In such a sleeping state can the practiser still breathe slowly to avoid drowsiness?

Answer He should slow down his breathing not only when he is in bed but also when sitting in meditation. Before so sitting he should loosen his clothes, breathe out impure and inhale fresh air in order to set his heart at rest. He should take the same mental attitude as when he sleeps, that is seeing and hearing nothing, close his mouth and touch the palate with the tip of the tongue, empty the mind of all thoughts, drive down the air breathed in and abstain from moving his limbs. He should then concentrate on spirit (between and behind the eyes) and drive it down into the cavity of vitality (under the navel) where spirit and vitality become inseparable, like slow fire kept in a stove. As time passes his spirit becomes stronger and he will even forget about sleeping; his vitality will be full and cause him to forget about eating; his generative force will be full freeing him from all sexual desires and causing his body to be strong and light; his heart will be pure and spiritual; his vitality will be genuine; his spirit will be perfect and divine; thus he will enter upon the path of immortality. This resting breath is far more advanced than the foetal breath.

Question You have said that the wheel of the law (the immortal breathing) is self-winding and that it does not turn if the practiser has not received authentic instruction from competent masters. Will you please tell my why?

Answer The wheel of the law is self-winding but since positive vitality cannot by itself leave its own cavity (under the navel) to rise and fall (in the microcosmic orbit), it should be driven by postnatal (vital) breath from the heels and mortal gate into the channels of control and function to go up to the head (heaven) and down to the lower abdomen (earth). The technique consists of using postnatal (vital) breath to set prenatal vitality in motion so that the wheel of the law can turn of itself.

When I was sixty, one day during my meditation I felt as if ants were running all over my body, and unexpectedly my lower tan t'ien centre (under the navel) became unusually hot and most relaxing overwhelming me with great joy. All of a sudden my penis stood up and my prenatal vitality vibrated causing my genital organ to retract. As I unconsciously refrained from loosening my grip on this vitality the latter was restrained by my genital organ as if to unite with it. At this stage vitality seemed to but actually did not drain away. Then positive vitality went down and veered to the base of the backbone to ascend slowly. Simultaneously the channels of control and function opened by themselves. I immediately practised immortal breathing through the heel and trunk pathways to turn the wheel of the law and the result achieved was so mysterious that it is beyond description.

If no indication is given to students, how can they practise and achieve this fourfold immortal breathing which is not by their nostrils or mouth? The question is whether or not they succeed in meeting competent masters, but who dares to divulge the great Tao which is so profound?

I have studied and practised alchemy until my seventy-third year and now undertake to reveal it in this book so that serious students can understand it properly within a short length of time.

10

THE METHOD OF GATHERING VITALITY

When (vital) breath vibrates and the penis stands erect, the practiser should press his middle fingers on the dragon and tiger cavities (in the centres of the two palms), raise his tongue to the palate to make a bridge linking with the channel of control, look up and to the left, breathe in to raise (vitality) to the region of the brain (ni wan) and then breathe out to lower it to the mortal gate (at the root of the penis). After several such ascents and descents, the genital organ will retract.

This is how to gather the generative force and vitality. To gather vitality is to insure its free circulation and to gather the generative force is to hold it in reserve for purification. By so doing the practiser will enjoy long life.

The generative force should be stored in full to guard against the loss of 'the precious thing' at night (by nocturnal emission). To achieve this the practiser should place the left palm on the right one, bending the two middle fingers to press on the dragon and tiger cavities (in the centres of his palms); raise the tongue to the palate to make a bridge linking with the channel of control; then breathe in to lift vitality up and breathe out to lower it in order to prevent the generative fluid from draining away. This is the method of holding up the generative force and vitality.

Chapter 9 teaches how to transmute the generative force and vitality into immortal seed but before the latter matures it tends to vibrate at night and drain away of itself even in the absence of thoughts and dreams. At this stage the practiser should be very careful. But how does he avoid nocturnal emission?

He should follow the method taught in this chapter to prevent the loss of the 'precious thing' in his sleep. If he has previously given rise to perverse thoughts while gathering the generative force, to sexual desires when seeing attractive women or to disturbance at licentious talk, the arousal of the genital organ indicates that he will lose the 'precious thing' at night even in the absence of thoughts during his sleep. It will be a matter for regret if he does not practise the method dealt with here to stop nocturnal emission.

One of my disciples who was seventy came to see me, weeping and saying: 'I have surmounted all difficulties in my practice but last night I failed to stop positive principle draining away; will you please teach me how to prevent its recurrence?'

I said: 'If you restart your training from the first step (Chapter I) to remedy this loss, you will still succeed later on, but if you do not start all over again, you will return home to wait for your death because there is no other method. When I gave you instruction, I told you that if the genital organ quivers, you should guard against the loss of positive principle at night and urged you to practise the tenth step (given in this chapter) to gather vitality. If you have disregarded my instruction and have now lost the positive principle, you can only blame yourself.' He said: 'My genital organ was aroused and quivered that day and

I intended to practise step ten that evening but after being kept busy the whole day with my house work I forgot everything at night; this was the cause of my trouble.'

I said: 'You are already in your seventieth year but disregard your (essential) nature and (eternal) life, to attend to house work. From now on every morning and evening you should train diligently with a mind set at rest during your sitting and forget all about your house work. Then concentrate both eyes pointedly on the lower tan t'ien centre (under the navel) and breathe deeply so that your breath reaches that centre. If you do this for one hundred days your lower tan t'ien will become hot, your eyes will flash light and you will hear something like wind blowing in your ears; you will thus restore the positive principle that has been dispersed. You should then practise microcosmic orbiting (by turning the wheel of the law) to repair the damage, doing it gently in order to avoid strain. If you so train you will certainly produce the immortal seed which, however, before it matures, tends to arouse and shake the penis without prior warning.

'Each evening before going to bed, relax your heart and sit in meditation. First locate the dragon cavity by bending the middle finger of your left hand and where it touches the left palm is that cavity which is lively and is linked with the heart and the lower abdomen by a channel (artery) passing through the left wrist. Then locate the tiger cavity by bending the middle finger of your right hand and where it touches the right palm is that cavity which also is linked with the heart and lower abdomen by a channel (vein) passing through the right wrist.

'Now place the right palm on the left pressing the right middle fingertip on the dragon cavity (in the left palm) and the left middle fingertip on the tiger cavity (in the right palm) thus blocking both cavities. Draw in the genital organ, shut the mouth, touch the palate with the tongue, breathe in through the nostrils while rising the eyes from the left to look up, and then breathe out while lowering the eyes to look down. This is turning the eyes to drive the (vital) breath up and down in the nostrils.

'After turning the eyes up and down nine times pause a little and draw in the genital organ as before.

'Repeat the same exercise for a second, third and fourth time to complete thirty-six turns of the eyes in order to block the channel of the generative and vital forces (at the mortal gate at the base of the penis). After so preventing nocturnal emission, practise the microcosmic orbiting to repair all deficiencies. When the generative and vital forces are fully recovered, prenatal vitality tends to escape by the anus causing you to break wind frequently. If this is due to gas in the stomach and intestines which comes from food and drink, it is good to let it escape by the anus, but if it is prenatal vitality it is most important to stop it.

'The Fa Chueh says: "Plug the dragon and tiger cavities (as taught above), raise the tongue to the palate to link the channels of control and function, contract the anus and look up and down to drive the (vital) breath (up and down) in the nasal channel seven times. This exercise will retain and spread prenatal vitality to all parts in the body in order to strengthen it; and thus the tendency to break wind will stop."

'If you are inconvenienced by the need to go to the lavatory more frequently than usual and if it is some way from your room, the best method is to plug the dragon and tiger cavities (in the palms), touch the palate with the tongue, contract the anus, look up and down to drive the (vital) breath (up and down) in the nose, contract the ducts of discharge (of urine and excrement), and you will get rid of the trouble.

'The above precaution is to prevent the drain of vitality without which the spiritual seed cannot develop. If the spiritual seed is defective how can you extinguish fire when it should be put out. If fire cannot be stopped at this stage it will be impossible to break through the great gate (of the original cavity of spirit in the centre of the brain). If this breakthrough is not achieved it will be impossible to stop the drain of vitality and to retract the genital organ; if so how can the immortal seed develop? Without the immortal seed how can the immortal foetus develop? Without the immortal foetus how can you leave the body through the heavenly gate (aperture of Brahma at the top of the skull) to become a heavenly immortal (t'ien hsien)?

'My, masters Liao Jan and Liao K'ung said: "Real Tao means spirit and vitality only. Cultivation of vitality is negative and of spirit is positive. When both the negative and the positive unite in one, the latter produces positive spirit which can manifest in bodily form visible to others, whereas negative spirit cannot manifest visibly."

'The ten steps taught up to here consist of uniting spirit and vitality to produce the immortal seed. Therefore, if pre-natal vitality drains away at night, how can the immortal seed be produced? If the genital organ is not aroused vitality will not drain away but when it is stirred and quivers by itself nocturnal emission is bound to occur in sleep.

'Therefore, before sleeping you should block the dragon and tiger cavities in the palms and do the exercise which I have explained.

'The accumulation of generative and vital forces in adequate quantity will automatically lead to the stage when fire is no longer needed and should be stopped (by no longer regulating the breathing) to produce the macrocosmic alchemical agent for the breakthrough. When you reach this stage, the practice of (turning the wheel of the law or) the microcosmic orbit technique (hsiao chou t'ien) is no longer needed.

'The ancients also mentioned the drain of positive vitality caused by the failure to stop fire in order to gather the macrocosmic alchemical agent, but in your case your genital organ is aroused and shaken by the evil fire (of passion) due to lack of vitality and the weakness of the alchemical agent; if you do not gather more vitality and block the discharge channel for the generative fluid you cannot prevent the positive principle draining away.'

Students should ponder over all this. When the generative force is full and the elixir is mature, the genital organ will not dilate and quiver and will draw in. If fire is not stopped when it is no longer needed it also causes nocturnal emission. These two different states should be clearly understood by all practisers.

The above method of gathering the generative and vital forces is for the purpose of producing the immortal seed. When enough of these forces is gathered there will be no nocturnal emission and no drain of vitality by the anus which should not be mistaken for breaking wind. If however vitality is being lost the practiser should block the dragon and tiger centres (in the palms) as already explained, raise the tongue to the palate to link it with the channel of control, drive the (vital) breath in and out while rolling the eyes to push vitality up the backbone and down the front part of the body. This exercise, done seven times, will divert from the anus vitality which will spread to all parts of the body to invigorate it. If there is frequent need to ease nature the practiser should contract the anus and wait for about half a day before going to the lavatory in order to prevent vitality from draining away so that it returns to its source (under the navel) and the immortal seed can form.

This is the method of gathering prenatal vitality to return it to its cavity (below the navel) to form the immortal seed.

My elder brother Chao K'uei I said:

When vitality drains because the penis swells and quiver
It should be turned back to its centre to strengthen the
body.
No means to realise essential nature
Can overlook both spirit and vitality.

The master Liu Ming Jui said:

When enjoying the taste of spring
Guard against risks to the body
By blocking the dragon and tiger cavities
'Til immortal seed breaks through the Great Barrier.

The master P'eng Mou Chang said:

Drive to the head vitality vibrating
And roll your eyes to control (vital) breathing
To cultivate the immortal seed by day
And night so that it rays out light from within the brain.

Question I have listened to your teaching on the ten steps (Chapters 1 to 10) but when my genital organ dilated and quivered in spite of my having blocked the drain of generative and vital forces by rolling my eyes to drive the breath in and out in the four stages of nine turns each, I failed to stop nocturnal emission. What is the reason?

Answer The outer agent which you have gathered is an illusory false one created by wrong thoughts; hence the nocturnal emission. This illusory agent is the generative fluid which contains the evil fire that develops when it is aroused by the vital force. The genital organ swells and quivers when the generative and vital forces vibrate causing this evil fire to scorch the testicles and so dilate the generative duct to drain the positive principle away. You have wrongly used this generative fluid which cannot be transmuted into immortal seed when it contains the evil fire (of passion) and cannot be employed to produce the macrocosmic agent; the most you can expect is to improve your health by eradicating all ailments. The correct method consists of using prenatal vitality, which is not produced by evil thoughts and which alone can be transmuted into immortal seed, to break through the Great Barrier (or Gate in the original cavity of spirit).

Question You have taught us to press the middle fingers on the dragon and tiger cavities (in the palms), raise the tongue to the palate, make pointed concentration to shrink the genital organ, drive the breath in and out of the nostrils and roll the eyes up and down in order to block the duct that discharges the generative force, but I do not think that the centres of the palms and the in and out breaths are linked with that channel and wonder how it can be blocked in order to prevent nocturnal emission. Will you please explain in detail?

Answer The channels conveying blood and vital force to the centres of the palms start from the heart. The channels conveying vitality to the left hand is an artery (called) the dragon; prenatal vitality coming from the heart passes through the wrist and carries blood to the centre of the left palm, which is the dragon cavity. The channel carrying blood and vitality from the right ventricle of the heart is a vein which is linked with the duct of the testicles and the restraining nerve; hence the centre of the right palm is the tiger cavity. When the dragon and tiger cavities are pressed with the middle fingers, the two channels to the heart and lower abdomen are blocked and their passage through the wrists is closed.

The heart is the seat of (essential) nature which manifests through the eyes while the lower abdomen is the seat of life which manifests through the genital organ.

In your practice to restrain and retract the genital organ, when you breathe in through the nose you actually lift the vital breath by turning your eyes up from the lower left, and when you breathe out you lower the vital breath by turning your eyes down from the upper right. You should realise that, since the heart is linked with the two eyes, this exercise in four phases of nine complete turns each causes vitality in the heart to restrain vitality in the tiger cavity while you look up to turn the eyes, and to shut the genital duct while you look up to lift the vital breath. If so how can the positive principle drain away?

Question When the heart is aroused and causes the penis to erect suddenly, is it because the genital root dilates and quivers?

Answer No, because the genital root dilates and vibrates in the state of thoughtlessness and unconsciousness; this is caused by vitality in the scrotum which stirs the testicles and widens the duct by which the generative fluid drains away. If you do not practise the tenth step (as described in this chapter) which consists of contracting the genital gate, you will be unaware of nocturnal emission which will continue and so nullify all previous progress; this is because of your carelessness.

As to the erection of the penis in the absence of (perverse) thoughts, this is due to the manifestation of the positive principle at the living hour of tsu (11 p.m.–1 a.m.) when you should take advantage of it to practise the two phases (of ascent and descent in the microcosmic orbit) in order to gather the alchemical agent (as explained earlier).

Therefore, you should not confound the dilation and vibration of the genital root with the erection of the penis for they have nothing in common.

Question You have said that the alchemical agent cannot be gathered if the genital root does not dilate and quiver at the living hour of tsu. I think the latter does so when vitality vibrates in the lower tan t'ien (under the navel) and that if it is not turned back there will be nocturnal emission of positive vitality. Will you please teach me what to do here?

Answer In your meditation when you achieve utter stillness the inner mechanism suddenly dilates and quivers in the absence of evil thoughts that stir the passionate heart. This is caused by the vibration of vitality in the lower tan t'ien centre (under the navel) in spite of the absence of thoughts. If the practiser does not recognise this vibrating vitality he will achieve nothing. When this happens, he should practise the ten steps (Chapters 1 to 10) to turn vitality back to nurture the immortal seed. His leap from the worldly to the saintly state will be made possible by (the proper use of) this shaking vitality which in sexual intercourse begets offspring. All things in the world are reproduced also through this vibrating vital force. The practiser of alchemy also uses it to produce the immortal seed.

My masters said: 'Immortality cannot be cultivated or attained unless sexual vitality vibrates. But heretics do not know the method of using this vitality.'

The ancient masters awaited this vibration and, instead of thinking about it, immediately practised the two phases of ascent and descent (as previously taught); by breathing in and out they turned vitality back to produce and nurture the immortal seed; this is the method of stopping nocturnal emission to prolong life. All this has nothing to do with sexual desires. However, if you give rise to lust while practising alchemy you will make a very, very grave mistake and I shall not accept you as my disciple. When vitality vibrates, if the practiser, for want of self-respect, gives rise to sexual desire, he will simply hasten the end of his life.

Question I have seen many old people and sickly youths die prematurely for want of self-respect. Is there a method to avoid such an untimely death?

Answer When the genital organ dilates and quivers some old people wrongly give rise to sexual desire and enjoy intercourse. If they fall ill because of the weather or unwholesome food there is nothing in their bodies to sustain their falling spirit and vitality and stop the drain of generative fluid. This is the cause of their untimely death. Most youths think they are young and strong and that death is still far away; so they let their generative and vital forces drain away until these are exhausted and their health declines; how then can they avoid premature death?

Old people who are weak should avail themselves of the arousal of vitality to act immediately even before turning away their perverse thoughts. They should concentrate on the mortal gate (at the root of the penis) and breathe in to lift (the vital force there) up to (the lower tan t'ien cavity which is) 1.3 inches under the navel, pause a little before concentrating on the chiang kung centre (or the solar plexus) and then breathe out to lower the vital force there to the cavity of vitality (under the navel). From there positive vitality will spread to all parts of the body, killing all sexual desires. This exercise is to be repeated until the genital organ shrinks. If they so train how can there be desire for sexual intercourse?

11

DRIVING THE ELIXIR OF IMMORTALITY INTO THE CAULDRON

1

When the spiritual foetus is formed by the ball of fire
A white light from the heart illuminates all
Things and a great blaze of golden light appears;
When all channels have been cleared the macrocosmic
     agent's made.

2

The bright pearl illuminates the brain
Making in nine turns the elixir.
Only when a drop sinks down to the belly
Does one realise immortals live on earth.

The above stanzas deal with the generative force, vitality and spirit which, after being sublimated, gather in the brain where, under constant pressure from prenatal vitality and spirit, they will in time produce ambrosia (kan lu). The latter flowing into the mouth becomes a liquid (saliva) which, when swallowed, makes 'sounds' in the abdomen. This ambrosia produces and nurtures the immortal seed in the lower tan t'ien (under the navel) whence it radiates, lighting up the heart. The light reveals the formation of the immortal seed when all breathing (appears to) cease and pulses to stop beating. This achievement is due mainly to the condition of utter stillness which contributes to the production of the immortal seed.

The cultivation of immortality does not go beyond spirit and vitality. Spirit leads to the realisation of (essential) nature and vitality to (eternal) life. Spirit comes from the sublimation of vitality and vitality from the purification of the generative force. To become immortal it is most important to sublimate the generative force, and when (refined) vitality is full it will manifest. If vitality is used to nurture the generative force the latter, when full, will produce the immortal seed.

All Taoist scriptures, in spite of the diversity of teaching, do not go beyond (essential) nature and (eternal) life. To discuss anything further leads to speculations that deceive and mislead the ignorant. You may speak in as many ways as you like but if you do not know the secrets of transforming the generative force into vitality, vitality into spirit and the return of spirit to the great emptiness, you will only formulate heresy. If you want to achieve immortality you must start by cultivating (essential) nature and (eternal) life, which will surely lead to the attainment of your goal.

This spirit is what the six first steps (Chapters 1 to 6) teach you to realise, that is the true light of (essential) nature in the cultivation of both nature and life; this light is spirit.

As to the light of vitality, it is what the six following steps (Chapters 7 to 12) teach you to realise, that is the light of (eternal) life in the cultivation of both nature and life; this light is vitality in the generative force.

The union of spirit and vitality produces the immortal seed as revealed by the white light in the heart, lights flashing in the head, the dragon's hum and the tiger's roar in the ears. If the light of ambrosia is not full and bright, this is due to lack of instruction and guidance by enlightened masters. In this event inner fire should be gathered and lifted to produce spiritual fire which will emit the golden light, and then the light of ambrosia will be full and bright. But you should not gather and lift fire at this stage for too long as it may cause dizziness. If the immortal seed is fully developed the golden light will manifest; if it does not further training is necessary (as follows):

Each day while sitting in meditation, the practiser should unite the two pupils (i.e. draw them together by squinting) to concentrate on and drive spirit and vitality into the lower tan t'ien (under the navel) in order to produce and nurture the immortal seed. When the latter is produced the practiser will feel as if the top of his head is raised; the dragon's hum and tiger's roar are heard in his ears;[1] his body floats on the clouds and itches all over; he rises in space and rides on the wind, with an accompanying sense of boundless bliss. He will then feel as if a spider's web covers his face or tickling ants swarm over it from his forehead to the bridge of the nose, eye sockets, cheeks, jaws, teeth and mouth causing continual secretion of saliva which cannot all be swallowed (in one gulp). He is now disinclined to open his mouth or move his body, thus falling into a state of indistinctness in which nothing seems to exist, even his own body cannot be found, his breathing (appears to) stop and his pulses (to) cease beating. Vitality is fully developed and nurtures the immortal seed. Hence it is said; 'Fullness of vitality makes the practiser forget all about eating.'

At this stage if he continues eating, the negative principle will remain and the positive principle will not be genuine and will arouse his appetite. As a result the immortal seed cannot form because of deficient vitality.

---

[1] The tiger's roar heard in the left ear reveals the fullness of vitality, and the dragon's hum in the right ear reveals the fullness of generative force.

The practiser should train until he achieves stillness and radiance of his spirit which, when full, will make him forget about sleeping. When his vitality is fully developed and enables him to dispense with eating, he reaches the stage of constant stillness and radiance in which breathing (appears to) cease and a massive golden light manifests while all discriminations stop arising, prior to his realisation of perfect serenity. This achievement is revealed by the moonlight appearing in the forehead which will remain constantly there if he is firmly determined to hold on to the original cavity of spirit (between and behind the eyes) while sparks appear between the eyebrows; both manifestations announce the full growth of the immortal seed.

Henceforth the practiser should guard against the drain of vitality in order to hold it in the body for nurturing and developing the immortal seed. During the latter's growth he should avoid the ten following excesses: 1, excessive walking which adversely affects his nerves; 2, standing, his bones; 3, sitting, his blood; 4, sleeping, his blood vessels; 5, listening, his generative force; 6, looking (at things), his spirit; 7, speaking, his breath; 8, thinking, his stomach; 9, sexual pleasure, his life; and 10, eating, his heart. In short he should avoid all excesses which are very harmful.

While sitting in meditation the practiser should never: 1, give rise to thoughts which cause the (inner) fire to flare up; 2, relax his concentration to avoid cooling down the (inner) fire; 3, look at external objects, for there the spirit wanders thereby harming the incorporeal soul (hun); 4, listen to outer sounds, for this scatters the generative force and so harms the corporeal soul (p'o); 5, breathe quickly, for such breaths disperse easily and cannot be regulated; and 6, break his breath rhythm, for its abrupt stoppage will make it weak when resumed; and when he suddenly stops breathing he cools his (vital) breath and when he starts again suddenly he heats it thereby damaging the immortal seed. If he does not pay attention to all this he will achieve nothing.

Therefore, when thoughts arise the practiser should use the inner fire that has flared up to turn the wheel of the law (i.e. direct it into the microcosmic orbit) to wipe them out, but he should never turn it when unsteady concentration has cooled down the inner fire so as not to injure the immortal seed. His eyes should not look at things but should be closed and turned back to gaze at the white light that appears between them; this is correct seeing. If he is stirred by sense data and opens his eyes to look outward, his concentration and spirit will scatter damaging the immortal seed. His ears should not listen to external sounds and voices because if his hearing is disturbed not only will his heart and body shake but also the immortal seed will be affected and scatter. He should not be impatient about forming the immortal seed because impatience will stir the heart and prevent the seed from developing. His training should take its natural course, that is it should be neither overlooked nor stressed. His awareness of spirit in the cavity of vitality (under the navel) should not be increased by the thought of holding it there, for unless he breathes naturally all the time he will never reach the state of indistinctness.

At this stage the genital organ will draw in but when its root dilates and shakes the practiser may mistake this as revealing the formation of the immortal seed. If the latter is mature he should stop the inner fire to gather the macrocosmic alchemical agent; if it is not he should take advantage of this vibration of vitality to turn the wheel of the law (i.e. the microcosmic orbit) to nurture that seed.

There is a method of knowing whether the immortal seed is mature or not which consists of placing an oil lamp in front of the practiser whose eyes should gaze at its flame while rolling them from left to right nine times, after which he closes them. If a great moonlight appears between the eyes, as bright as the glare of lightning which neither increases nor contracts, the immortal seed is mature. If he sees a circle whose centre is obscure and border bright, the seed is immature; in this event further training is necessary.

The above method is to raise the inner fire to arouse spiritual fire so that the golden light appears. It should not be practised frequently in order to avoid dizziness and waste of vitality that radiates, for the aim of the practice is to realise this prenatal vitality and also the manifestation of this light which is spirit that lies between (and behind) the two eyes. For the ultimate goal of thousands of methods of practice does not go beyond the realisation of vitality and spirit.

During my meditation under the guidance of my masters Liao Jen and Liao K'ung, I practised the ten steps to build up the generative and vital forces in sufficient quantities and then to transmute the generative force into its prenatal form of vitality in order to produce the immortal seed. During each daily sitting I drew the pupils of my eyes close together to concentrate on my lower abdomen until I felt something like itching over my face, a spider's web covering it and a swarm of ants crawling over it; this showed that prenatal vitality pervaded all parts of my body. The dragon's hum and tiger's roar were in my ears, and more saliva gathered than I could swallow (in one gulp). Then suddenly I sank into a state of indistinctness wherein my consciousness and awareness of things seemed to vanish. My body seemed to roam on the top of the clouds. This revealed prenatal vitality that nurtured and developed the immortal seed.

This seed is immature if it contains negative breath and mature if free of it. When it matures the practiser does not want to sleep and when prenatal vitality is full he does not want to eat. At this stage when he breathes in and out through the nostrils or mouth, no outside air (appears to) enter or leave by them. Then a white light appears constantly in front of him and his body cannot be found anywhere.

This is the preliminary stage of serenity in which he should guard against nocturnal emission that drains his generative force. He should avoid strain and overwork by day because if he is too tired the positive principle will drain away at night. He should rest by sitting in meditation in order to nurture and develop the immortal seed as his main objective. He should avoid inquiring into anything so that his ears hear nothing and his heart (the house of fire) is disengaged from all sense data. If thoughts arise inadvertently he should immediately turn the wheel of the law, close and turn back his eyes to gaze at the light of immortal seed, then rising thoughts will disappear automatically. While dwelling in this thoughtless state he should look into the lower tan t'ien centre (under the navel) in which a gentle breath fans the vitality. The latter becomes hot and from it the light of the elixir will rise so that the whole space between the navel and the eyes is filled with a white light. The root of the genital organ will then vibrate and he may wrongly think that the immortal seed is mature but it is not. He should take advantage of the vibration to gather the alchemical agent to nurture that seed.

In order to know if the seed is mature or not, he should follow the method previously mentioned by placing an oil lamp in front of him and looking at its flame while rolling his eyes round from left to right nine times; if he then closes them and sees a great white light surrounded by lightning-like sparks, the immortal seed is mature. If he sees a dark circle surrounded by sparks, the seed is immature; in this event he should gather the alchemical agent to develop that light, and then practise once more the twelve steps (taught in this book).

This is called raising and lifting the inner fire to produce spiritual fire in order to see if the seed is fully developed but do not do this too often or it will cause dizziness and harm the generative force, vitality and spirit.

The master P'eng Mou Chang said: 'The method of producing the immortal seed consists of "uniting" the heart with the eyes for pointed concentration on the lower abdomen so that if vibration is felt there, vitality can be immediately circulated (in the microcosmic orbit) for purification, but the slightest carelessness on the part of the practiser can cause it to drain away thereby nullifying all previous progress.

'If at this preliminary stage the genital organ shrinks this does not prove that it is really drawn in. If the immortal seed only sparks it is immature. The practiser should continue to work diligently until the penis (appears to) shrink into the lower abdomen. A white light will first appear in front of the eyebrows and, as time passes, will fill the space between them and the lower tan t'ien (under the navel); this reveals the maturity of the immortal seed. But if after long training this light fails to appear the practiser should light and place an incense stick before him, and then focus his eyes to gaze at its burning tip; after rolling them round from left to right nine times, the immortal seed will be completely mature and bright. Further training is needed to lift this bright light of the elixir from the lower tan t'ien (under the navel) to the eyes which will then flash two or three times. This light of the elixir glitters like pure gold and resembles a ball of fire which is a sign that the immortal seed is fully developed.'

The old master Liu Yun P'u said: 'The practiser should know the method of nurturing and developing the immortal seed. If the spirit is not serene the seed cannot form and the elixir of immortality cannot be prepared. If (vital) breath is not held in the lower tan t'ien the light of the seed does not appear.

Both heart (house of fire) and breath should be frozen in the lower tan t'ien; although the (vital) breath may leave it occasionally, the heart should never stray from it. The heart and the pupils of the eyes should always concentrate on that centre until the postnatal (vital) breaths return and stay there to sustain prenatal vitality which will nurture and develop the seed that causes the light of the elixir to manifest. The latter is like a ball of fire, the size of a bullet, in the lower tan t'ien centre which will become hot causing the root of the genital organ to vibrate and set prenatal vitality in motion. The practiser should now visualise this vitality as rising from the base of the spine in the channel of control (tu mo) up to the ni wan or brain, thence descending (by the channel of function) to the mortal gate (at the base of the penis) to spread to all parts of the body and limbs. As a result vitality and blood will become all-pervading, invigorate the body and nurture and develop the immortal seed.'

The immortal T'an Chih Ming said: 'The great Tao consists of sublimating the generative force into vitality whose fullness will nurture and develop the immortal seed, the light of which reveals the real positive generative force. This is the cultivation of both (essential) nature and (eternal) life, the object of which is to realise full development of positive vitality. If spirit wavers causing nocturnal emission of the 'most precious thing' the absence of this light confirms the loss of real positive generative force. All students should pay particular attention to this sublimating method for if the immortal seed is properly nurtured within, it will sustain the positive generative force without, causing the light of (essential) nature and (eternal) life to manifest.'

The Nan Hua Ching says: 'The real positive generative force is mysterious.' The Tao Te Ching says: 'The generative force which is real, exists within that which is profound and mysterious.' This real generative force is the true seed in the human body. Since it is indistinct, it is called t'ai chi (the supreme ultimate) and since it is the beginning of creativity, it is called prenatal (hsien t'ien). Since it is the undivided yin-yang (the union of the negative and the positive) it is called the One vitality. It is also called the yellow bud (huang ya), the mysterious pearl (hsuan chu) and positive generative force (yang ching). If this generative force is frozen between heaven (the head) and earth (the lower abdomen) it becomes the light of immortal seed.

Question You have said that if the practiser has not received instruction from competent masters, the inner light which he may produce will not be full and bright. Will you explain why?

Answer It is called the light of vitality (hui kuang) and when it develops fully it is called the golden light (shan kuang). The generative force which is still immature cannot produce the white light of vitality and the immortal seed which is immature cannot produce the golden light. The light of vitality is like the moon and the golden light (of the seed) shines like pure gold.

The immortal seed is the crystallisation of positive generative force. When the latter is fully developed the practiser should turn back his eyes to concentrate on and look into the lower tan t'ien centre (under the navel) so that the element of fire in the eyes which are above scorches that of water in the belly which is below, to produce positive vitality whose light manifests in front of him. The fullness of the generative force manifests as the white light of vitality and the fullness of the immortal seed as a golden light which reveals negative vitality within the generative force. The light of the eyes directed downward is positive and when the positive and negative lights meet, a precious light (pao kuang) will emerge.

This is like an electric current which, when the positive and negative poles are joined, gives a bright light, unless the power supply is deficient. In the same way unless the generative force has been fully restored to its strength at puberty it cannot produce the light of vitality which is white like moonlight.

When the generative force has been restored in full and becomes as effective as at puberty, which is revealed when the genital organ draws in, both positive and negative vitalities unite to produce a bright golden light which shines like pure gold. The white light of vitality reveals the imperfect body containing the negative principle which can produce earthly states while the golden light reveals the fullness of generative force, vitality and spirit which unite into a whole.

Any dimness in the light of vitality and in the golden light is caused by nocturnal emission of the 'precious thing'. This is likened to a short circuit that causes a blackout. If the electric bulb is broken, air will enter it and the light goes out. Likewise, if thoughts are allowed to arise during the meditation, outside air will enter the body and blow out the precious light. Students should pay particular attention to all this.

Question You have said that the practice of gathering and lifting fire to produce spiritual fire so that the golden light manifests, should not be repeated often as it causes dizziness and dissipates prenatal vitality. Will you please explain why?

Answer The organ of nature (hsin ken or the heart) is linked with the cavity of life (ming ch'iao or the lower tan t'ien under the navel) by a channel called the ch'ung ch'iao or ch'ung mo MNOA (see *figure 8* overleaf). When the (exhausted) generative force has been fully restored by the alchemical process, it will have access to the ocean of (essential) nature (hsin hai); this is the (tsu ch'iao) cavity in the centre of the brain which is linked with the two eyes and also with the heart (see pages 10-12). If in spite of this connection the precious light does not manifest at the early stage of practice, it is because the centre of (essential) nature (i.e. the tsu ch'iao) is still closed.

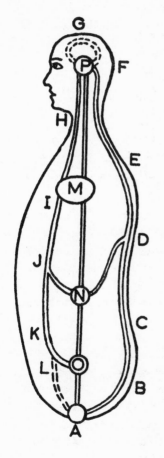

The channel of control (tu mo)
A B C D E F:
A (tzu *cardinal point North* –
the mortal gate (sheng szu
ch'iao)
B (ch'uo) intermediate point
C (yin) intermediate point
D (mao) *cardinal point East,*
wood (cleansing)
E (ch'en) intermediate point
F (szu) intermediate point
The channel of function (jen mo)
G H I J K L:
G (wu) *cardinal point South* –
the brain (ni wan)
H (wei) intermediate point
I (shen) intermediate point
J (ju) *cardinal point West,* metal
(purifying)
K (shu) intermediate point
L (hai) intermediate point
The thrusting channel (ch'ung
mo) M N O A:
M (li) the heart – house of fire
N (chung t'u) the central
earth, the solar plexus (chiang
kung)
O (k'an) the lower tan t'ien –
house of water
P The centre of the brain (tsu
ch'iao)

Figure 8 The channels of control, function and thrusting.

In order to open this centre of (essential) nature the practiser should place an oil lamp in front of him and concentrate his eyes on its flame, rolling them from left to right nine times to vibrate the (positive) vitality in that centre (between and behind the eyes) so that it drops to the cavity of (eternal) life (under the navel) already full of (negative) vitality so that both vitalities unite to thrust open the original cavity of spirit (tsu ch'iao in the centre of the brain). This is called the breakthrough of the original cavity from which the precious light emerges.

This light is bright like that of the moon, revealing the fullness of generative force and is called the light of vitality. When this light turns golden and glitters like pure gold, revealing the maturity of immortal seed, it is called golden light. If the centres at F and G are not linked the turning of the eyes will join them up. If the centres at L and A are not linked the process of sublimating vitality at D and J will join them up.

The technique of lifting fire should on no account be used frequently for to do so causes dizziness and injures vitality. Each turn of the eyes causes vitality in the cavity of life to soar up, spreading to the mouth, eyes, ears and nostrils which are the seven openings by which vitality scatters away. Of the seven, the heavenly pool cavity (t'ien ch'ih) above the mouth is the opening by which the greatest quantity of vitality drains away. This is why the loss of vitality due to excessive speaking and singing is comparatively greater than in other activities. Hence all practisers of Taoist meditation always touch the palate with the tip of the tongue whether they walk, stand, sit or recline, not only to block the heavenly pool and prevent the drain of vitality, but also to make a bridge by which vitality descends from the hsuan ying centre (the mysterious bridle behind the heavenly pool in the palate) down the throat, heart (M), chiang kung cavity (solar plexus) (N), lower tan t'ien centre (0), and mortal gate (A) to nurture the immortal seed.

All students should know that in the upper part of the body if the cavity of the heavenly pool (in the palate) is not blocked the hsuan ying cannot open; that in the lower part of the body if the channel of function (jen mo) is not blocked the control channel (tu mo in the spine) cannot open; and that in the middle part of the body if the other six channels (ch'ung mo, tai mo, yang ch'iao, yin ch'iao, yang wei and yin wei)[2] are not blocked, the cavity of spirit (between and behind the eyes) will not open and the vitality in the immortal foetus cannot come out.

When writing the above paragraph I could not refrain from tears (for it is not easy for students to meet enlightened masters). I have endured all sorts of difficulties and hardships in my search for well over thirty masters of whom only a few were truly enlightened whereas the majority were incompetent. This shows that it is not easy to find the authentic teachings which I now present in this book. If readers peruse it they will acquire in a short time the secrets of alchemy.

[2]See note 1 on page 24 for detailed description of the eight psychic channels.

12

PREPARING THE ELIXIR OF IMMORTALITY

The deficiency of the immortal seed can be remedied by the use of slow and quick fires (from regulating the breathing) so that the genital organ will draw in, the inner light will manifest before the eyes, the dragon's hum and tiger's roar will be heard in the ears, and the heart (the house of nature) will be luminous. When the practiser is aware of the maturity of the immortal seed, he should stop the fire (by no longer regulating the breathing) to gather the macrocosmic alchemical agent for the final breakthrough (i.e. forcing open the original cavity of spirit between and behind the eyes, which will emit the precious light).

After the practiser has experienced all the six states mentioned in the last chapter as well as flashes of light and the retraction of his genital organ, he may not be able to gather anything when his penis suddenly stands as usual at the living hour of tsu (11 p.m.–1 a.m.) because the generative force and vitality are uniting to produce the immortal seed. In this case he should use the method of nurturing and developing the immortal seed, which consists of 'uniting' (squinting) and directing his two eyes to look into the lower tan t'ien centre (under the navel) to transmute his (essential) nature in its (rudimentary) state of (vital) breath into an entitative state; henceforth there will be only one harmonious vitality which will unite all imperfect breath and vitality in the body into one uniform whole which will manifest from the chest as uniform white moonlight within and without the practiser.

In this state of genial springtime real breath seems to exist and prenatal spirit becomes perceptible while vitality develops unceasingly. The practiser now should guard against the arousal of intellect which will prevent vitality from developing and spirit from continuing; he should never break the prohibition against both (utter) neglect and (undue) attention. If stirring thoughts cause the spiritual body to vanish, this is due to neglect; and if the heart does not wander outside and never strays from the spiritual body, this is due to absence of neglect. If he is unduly specific and obstinate thereby hindering the process of alchemy this is because of excessive attention; but if he refrains from interfering with what is happening quietly, this is freedom from undue attention. Neglect leads to dullness and confusion and excessive attention to the dissipation (of spirit and vitality); these are grave mistakes which all practisers should avoid.

The (vital) breath that disperses in all parts in the body is the dying breath; if it is held fast there is life but if it disperses life comes to an end; hence either mortality or immortality in the twinkling of an eye.

At this stage, when the foundation has been laid with all centres (and channels) cleared and no obstructions remaining, if the practiser is not strongly supported by a dogged determination, gives rise to passion when seeing beautiful forms, and lets spirit chase after sense data, once he slips, all previous progress will be fruitless. It is like upsetting the contents of a basket by turning it upside down.

The generative force is neither matter nor form; when it remains in the body, it is vitality and when it is discharged, it is the generative fluid. It is impaired within by the seven passions (i.e. joy, anger, grief, fear, love, hate and desire) that affect the heart and without by the ten harmful excesses and nine unsettled breaths. It spreads in all nerves, blood vessels and psychic channels in the body. If it is turned back from its earthly course, it can be gathered and returned to its original cavity (below the navel), and immortality can be attained.

The seven passions that damage vitality are: intense delight that harms the heart; intense anger the liver; grief the lungs; fear the gall bladder; love spirit; hate the disposition; and intense desire the stomach.

The ten excesses that injure vitality are: excessive walking that harms the nerves; standing the bones; sitting the blood; sleep the pulses; joy the generative force; looking (at things) the spirit; speaking the breath; thinking the stomach; eating the heart; and too much sex the life.

The nine unsettled breaths are caused by: anger which lifts and fear which lowers the breath; joy which slows it down; grief which disperses it; terror which throws it out of gear; thinking which ties it up; toil which wastes it; cold which collects and heat which scatters it.

If the practiser wishes to gather the macrocosmic alchemical agent for the final breakthrough he should guard against these seven passions, ten excesses and nine disorderly breaths. If he does not gather that agent for the final breakthrough but merely practises the other methods that follow the twelve steps already taught, he can prolong and enjoy his life.

Those who can gather the microcosmic alchemical agent but do not know how to practise or to sublimate it by fire by stages, waste their efforts because of the seven passions and sexual attractions arising from colour, form, carriage, speech (voice), softness (smoothness) and features; how then can they realise immortality?

Some study the stages of purification by fire and expect to achieve immortality, but they do not realise that this use of fire is like growing flowers in the winter; too much heat will shrivel and destroy the plants, while if it is weak they will not flower and bear fruit. The fire must not be too strong or too weak but just right. It is the same when you practise the sublimation by fire by stages, for if you do so correctly you are certain to produce the immortal seed.

Question What is the immortal seed, how does one produce it and know whether or not it is mature?

Answer When the generative force rises to unite with (essential) nature, the (white) light of vitality manifests; it is like moonlight and its fullness is equivalent to one half of a whole. When vitality descends to unite with (eternal) life, the golden light will manifest; it is a reddish yellow and its fullness is equivalent to the other half. The union of these two lights will produce that whole which is the immortal seed.

After the 'spiritual gem' has returned to its source (in the lower abdomen) a pointed concentration on it will, in time, cause a golden light to appear in the white light between the eyebrows. This is the embryo of the immortal seed produced by the union of the generative force, vitality and spirit into one whole. When the body is full of it within, light will manifest without. These white and golden lights are like the positive and negative ends of an electric wire; and the union of generative force, vitality and spirit is like the current without which there is no light. In the same way if the two lights have not mingled within there will be no illumination without. Their union is caused by having mingled the five (vital) breaths (see below) into one vitality to nurture the immortal seed in the lower abdomen. Without the intermingling of these five breaths the golden light will not manifest.

These breaths come from the vitality in the lower tan t'ien cavity (beneath the navel) from which they spread to the five viscera: to the lungs as the vital breath of the element of metal; to the heart as the vital breath of the element of fire; to the liver as the vital breath of the element of wood; to the stomach as the vital breath of the element of earth; and to the lower abdomen as the vital breath of the element of water. These five breaths may be either strong or weak but if they are too strong or too weak they cause illnesses and if they clog the respective viscera they cause paralysis and beriberi.

When the training causes all five vital breaths to return to the source (under the navel), vitality becomes active there and circulates (in the body) rising from the base of the backbone to the top of the head and reflecting the silvery light of the (spinal) marrow; it then drops to the throat and the viscera increasing its brightness like a full moon shining in the heart. If the element of fire is strong in the heart it will scorch the blood; so the practiser should avoid excessive talking and thinking to rest his heart. This restfulness will invigorate spirit and body, for spirit withers in disturbance and thrives in still-ness; it develops in (unlimited) voidness and weakens in (ob-structive) form.

Question What are the six states which show that the immortal seed is complete?

Answer When a golden light appears in the eyes, the back of the head vibrates audibly, the dragon's hum is heard in the right and the tiger's roar in the left ear, fire blazes in the lower tan t'ien centre (under the navel), bubbles rise in the body, spasms shake the nose, and the genital organ draws in. These are signs that the immortal seed is complete.

1 The golden light in the eyes reveals the light of (essential) nature which illumines the lower tan t'ien (under the navel), and will in time become golden to show the fullness of the luminous generative force, vitality and spirit.

2 The dragon's hum shows the fullness of vitality in the generative force. When vitality fills the tiny channels of the nervous (and psychic) systems, it produces indistinct sounds.

3 The tiger's roar is the sound of fully developed vitality which is active.

4 The audible vibration at the back of the head reveals the strength of fire in the generative force, vitality and spirit: it differs from the wrong type of fire which causes buzzing in the ears.

5 The blazing fire in the lower tan t'ien cavity (under the navel) which scorches the kidneys, comes from the fullness of the generative force and vitality from which it arises; careless-ness on the part of the practiser may cause nocturnal emission of the 'precious thing' for there is danger when fuel is so close to a fire.

6 As to the retractile genital organ, it shrinks back like that of a baby in the mother's womb, which comes out when he cries at birth. Before it retracts, that is when the training is not yet completely successful, fire should not be stopped.

Thus the six signs reveal the appropriate moment to stop fire (by no longer regulating the breathing), which is the *first* thing to do at this stage.

Question After practising the twelve steps taught by you, when the golden light appears, what should we do next?

Answer Pass all your time concentrating your eyes on the lower tan t'ien centre (under the navel) until the cavity of (essential) nature (in the heart) emits sparks of fire in the eyes. Watch (all this) quietly until in this long state of stillness these sparks produce a golden glow which is the first manifestation of positive light.

At this stage you should be provided with the four necessities of alchemy: utensils, money, companions and a suitable place (in which to meditate).

The utensils are: a round wooden object like a bun, covered with cotton, to sit on to block the anus; and a clothes-peg to close the nostrils.

Money is to buy food for the practiser and his companions.

Companions are friends also practising alchemy.

The place is a quiet hut or temple which is not too far from towns and cities.

Only after acquiring these four necessities can one leave for the mountain to practise the last steps. If one of them is lacking he should not practise the method of stopping fire; he can, however, gather the (microcosmic) alchemical agent to prolong his life while waiting for an opportunity to continue his training.

Question Will you please teach me the method of stopping fire so that when I have been provided with the four necessities, I can go to the mountain to continue the training?

Answer After the first manifestation of positive fire as explained above, the practiser should obtain the four necessities and go to a quiet place where he should continue to maintain the union of the lights of (essential) nature and (eternal) life. As time passes the golden light will suddenly reappear much brighter; this is the second manifestation of positive light. He should now practise (the method of) stopping fire to gather the macrocosmic alchemical agent. The third manifestation of positive fire will be quite different from the first two.

To stop fire means to stop (regulating the) breathing and circulating (vital) air which should now be replaced by the heart, spirit and thought which combine to go up by the channel of control (tu mo in the spine) and down by the channel of function (jen mo). He should not, however, neglect the inner heat for a moment, since to do so cools the vitality which should be constantly concentrated upon to keep it warm.

The practiser's companions should serve him with food and drink so that he can continue his training (without unnecessary worries).

As time passes demonic states will occur to the practiser in the form of visions of paradise in all its majesty with beautiful gardens and pools, or of hells with frightful demons with strange and awesome heads and faces constantly changing their hideous forms. If he is unable to banish these apparitions caused by the five aggregates as well as the visions of women and girls which disturb him, he must compose his heart (mind) which should be clear within and without. The correct method is not to see all that is visible nor hear all that is audible, but to concentrate intently on the inmost, to fix on the spot between them (the eyes) and to practise the seventh step (Chapter 7) to drive vitality through the four cardinal points A, D, G, and J (see page 84). This will remove all demonic hindrances instantly.

You should know that these hindrances are caused by negative (vital) breaths remaining in the viscera. Since the practiser now feels that negative breaths are strong whereas positive ones are still weak, he should now roll his eyes to let in the latter while driving away the former in order to remove all obstructions which will then vanish. Such obstructions are caused by perverse thoughts rising in the heart (mind) which change positive into negative (vital) breaths and prevent the three positive lights from manifesting and the macrocosmic alchemical agent from developing. This immature agent cannot produce a wholly positive body to achieve the final breakthrough.

My master Liao K'ung said: 'At the first manifestation of positive light, you should immediately provide yourself with the four necessities (for advanced training). When it manifests for the second time, you should at once stop the fire to produce the macrocosmic alchemical agent. When it manifests for the third time, you should immediately gather the macrocosmic agent to achieve the breakthrough in order to transmute vitality into spirit thereby leaping over the worldly to the saintly state, and so leaving the state of serenity to appear in countless transformation bodies.' The final achievement is made possible by the breakthrough as the main step.

Question Will you please explain in detail these three manifestations of positive fire?

Answer If after stopping the fire, the practiser does not know the above method of gathering the macrocosmic alchemical agent, the positive fire will not manifest for the third time. If he has received authentic instruction from a competent master and knows how to gather the agent immediately after stopping the fire, positive vitality in the lower tan t'ien centre (under the navel) will cause the immortal seed to radiate.

Since the light of (essential) nature in the original cavity of spirit (tsu ch'iao, between and behind the eyes) is now concentrated below the navel, the positive light of vitality in the latter centre will soar up to manifest before the eyes, thereby causing both lights to unite and remain constant, while the space between the eyes and the navel will emit sparks of red golden light. These two lights are like the male and female organs of a flower, the union of which will bear fruit. The following diagram shows the field of concentration for gathering the macrocosmic alchemical agent with the manifestation of positive light.

The method consists of constantly nurturing and preserving the two lights of nature and life by keeping them warm in the body. When they are fully developed, they will unite

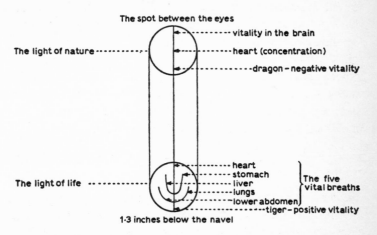

Figure 9 The field of concentration for gathering the macrocosmic alchemical agent.

automatically and will *never* scatter to form shapeless external light. At this stage the practiser feels as if his nasal breathing has ceased and his pulses have stopped beating, which reveals the fullness of (eternal) life after all twigs have returned to the root.

The reason for concentrating in the head the vital breaths (in the heart, stomach, liver, lungs and lower abdomen) is to gather the macrocosmic alchemical agent for the final breakthrough.

The Hui Ming Ching Chi Shuo says: 'When the light, whether white or golden, manifests to reveal (essential) nature, the practiser should call on a competent master and seek his instruction on gathering it. If it is not concentrated it will scatter, and he will miss a rare chance for the light will not reappear.

The method of gathering this light consists of rolling the eyes from A to D, G and J (see page 84). After it has been collected, the practiser should gather the macrocosmic alchemical agent after the six organs have shaken. If he does not the immortal seed cannot rise to the head and the final breakthrough cannot be achieved.

The practiser is now nearer his goal and should take the last step.

13

GATHERING THE MACROCOSMIC ALCHEMICAL AGENT FOR THE FINAL BREAKTHROUGH

This method consists of sitting in silent meditation to drive spirit and vitality into the lower tan t'ien centre (under the navel). The practiser should sit on a round piece of wood (the size of a small bun and covered with cotton) to block the mortal gate *below* thereby stopping vitality from draining away by the anus while the nostrils *above* should be closed with a clothes-peg to prevent the immortal seed from escaping by the nose. While dwelling in this bright stillness, he should avoid all strain and take advantage of the vibration of vitality to further and sustain the ascent of the macrocosmic alchemical agent which will then go up by itself in this state of mental indifference, but should on no account be driven up intentionally.

He should then practise the methods of 'the five dragons upholding the holy one', of 'driving the three vehicles uphill' and of 'sucking, pressing, pinching and shutting' which, if effectively performed, will produce the macrocosmic alchemical agent within six, instead of seven, days as mentioned in the books. This agent cannot be gathered in the absence of the foretelling states, and if the practiser is not provided with the four necessities mentioned earlier.

The six foretelling states which manifest when the macrocosmic alchemical agent is fully developed as explained in Chapter 12, do not all appear simultaneously on the same day. First, heat develops in the lower tan t'ien cavity (under the navel) after which the kidneys become hot like boiling water. Then the eyes reveal their golden mechanism. After that the tiger's roar is heard in the left and the dragon's hum in the right ear. Then the back of the head vibrates, bubbles rise in the body and spasms shake the nose. These are foretelling states pointing to the production of the macrocosmic alchemical agent, and are followed by the withering of the root of lust (in the testicles) and the accompanying transmutation of generative force into full vitality. When the latter vibrates, it will crystallize into the immortal seed and only then can the genital organ shrink as in babyhood. This is the real retractile state when the penis shrinks back and will no longer stand erect, causing the generative gate to shut and so preventing vitality from draining away. The practiser will thus achieve immortality.

The method of blocking the generative gate (at the tip of the penis) as previously taught is only to prevent vitality from draining away in order to preserve life. Hence the patriarch Li Hsu An said: 'Block it and again block it and only then can immortality be achieved; if it is not blocked (twice) immortality cannot be attained.' Therefore, seekers of immortality should pay special attention to this point.

When the generative gate is blocked for the second time, this is achieved by effective training which causes it to shut of itself. When this happens, the penis will no longer erect; and there will be no more generative force left to be sublimated. This is the proper time to stop fire (produced by regulated breathing) so that all the generative force which has been purified and accumulated in the testicles can now be transformed into the immortal seed.

When the golden light of this immortal seed manifests for the first time before his eyes, the practiser should immediately provide himself with the four necessities such as the required implements, provisions, companions and a quiet place for advanced training. If he is young and has parents and children to look after, he cannot retire to the mountain to train for the breakthrough and final leap over the worldly; he is, however, an earthly seer enjoying long life and freedom from all ailments. If his parents have died, his children have grown up and are independent, and he has no dependents to look after, he should provide himself quickly with these four necessities.

By implements are meant objects used during his advanced training, such as the wooden bun (to sit on) and the clothes-peg; by provisions an adequate supply for three to nine years; by companions those undergoing the same training and vowing to help him achieve the ultimate goal; and by a quiet place an ancient Taoist temple on some retired mountain far away from inhabited towns and silent cemeteries where negative influences obtain. It is advisable to choose an ancient abode where previous masters have realised immortality so that it is free from disturbing demons and the practiser can enjoy spiritual protection from his enlightened predecessors.

The immortal seed in the testicles is nurtured by positive vitality, and only when the latter has returned to its source (the lower tan t'ien centre under the navel) does the golden light appear for a second time.

After the second manifestation of the golden light, the positive vitality, now full, will replace the weakening (vital) breath to develop further. In the event of the breath vibrating, the practiser should gather the alchemical agent in full measure to repair the loss of generative force in order to restore its original fullness at puberty.

For the purpose of stopping fire, this gathering of the agent is not by breathing in and out but by concentrating the heart, spirit and thought on raising the agent in the backbone and lowering it down the front of the body so that the immortal seed develops fully. Suddenly sparks appear between the eyebrows, the heart is full of light, and vitality gives off a golden light which appears for the third time, which is the propitious moment to gather the macrocosmic alchemical agent.

The second manifestation of positive light is the signal to stop fire in order to gather the macrocosmic alchemical agent; its third is the signal to grasp the agent for the breakthrough. Its fourth manifestation will reveal the practiser's failure to stop the fire by his wrong use of in and out breaths at this stage, for the agent will follow (the fire which has not been stopped) to drain away in the form of postnatal generative fluid, thereby nullifying all progress so far achieved. Students are urged to pay particular attention to all this.

As to the method of gathering the macrocosmic alchemical agent within seven days for the final breakthrough, it consists of daily (constant) concentration of the two eyes on the lower tan t'ien centre (under the navel) so that, as time passes, the six foretelling states will manifest. The practiser should use the method of shaking the six sense organs to arouse the immortal seed so that it will pass through the three gates (in the backbone).

The six sense organs are: the nose, genital organ, eyes, ears, tongue and intellect. Their vibrations originate from the intellect which stirs the nose and tongue with an in breath which also affects the ears and eyes. As a result the genital organ vibrates arousing the immortal seed which then becomes very active. When the six sense organs vibrate, the immortal seed in the testicles will move to the mortal gate (at the root of the penis) which is shut but will, however, pass through it to thrust upward to the heart where it is blocked in the 'thrusting channel' (ch'ung mo – see *figure 8* on page 141) which is not open. It then moves down to enter the channel of control (tu mo) but the base of the spine is not open.

If the practiser does not know the methods of *'five dragons upholding the holy one'*, of *'sucking, pressing, pinching and shutting'* and of *'spirit lifting the goat cart'* the immortal seed will not follow the correct path and will veer from the (unopen) base of the spine to find an outlet through the anus which is a natural opening by which to drain away; if so all previous progress will be wasted. This is the danger of a fall from the lower magpie bridge (hsia ch'ueh ch'iao, the anus).

This is why the two immortals Ts'ao and Ch'iu devised a small round piece of wood with a convex top of the size of a (small Chinese) bun (man t'ou) and covered with cotton to sit on in order to *close* the anus and so prevent the macrocosmic alchemical agent from scattering away. If in addition a companion is available to help by *pinching* the base of the spine[1] the macrocosmic alchemical agent will enter and rise up in the channel of control (tu mo in the backbone).

We now know that the macrocosmic alchemical agent will remain stationary if its passage through the coccyx is blocked. If it is pushed through the base of the spine as willed by the practiser, this heterodox intention to lift it will fail for the least stir in the heart (the house of fire) at this stage will automatically close the coccyx. Hence the method of *'five dragons upholding the holy one'* is devised to accelerate its passage.

---

[1]If the practiser is alone and has no one to help him he can employ another method which consists of rubbing with his own hands the lower part of the backbone *down* to its base to warm the marrow above the coccyx in order to draw the agent up. Rubbing should always be *downward* but never upward; this is the most important point which all practisers should keep constantly in mind.

Although the passage of the 'precious gem' is blocked and although neither stir in the heart (the seat of the fire of passion) nor concentration of spirit can set it moving, the companion's *pinch* warms and loosens the marrow in the coccyx (to let it pass). In addition, the practiser should also *press* a finger on the mortal gate (at the root of the penis), and vitality in the precious gem will by itself thrust through the base of the spine.

Therefore, the practiser should not concentrate on pushing the agent to set it moving but should wait for it to thrust of itself and then gently guide it into the right channel. When it suddenly moves to thrust into the coccyx the practiser should assist it by pressing a finger on the mortal gate, raising his eyes at the same time to help it up. Then he should gently and slowly roll his eyes once acting like a *goat slowly drawing a cart uphill* in order to help the agent in its ascent. He should also support this ascent by *pressing* his tongue against the palate and *sucking* in a breath through the nose. Finally if he stretches the small of the back with a crack, the agent will of itself thrust into the base of the spine (the first gate in the backbone).

Now his companion should immediately *pinch* the backbone above the coccyx to further the gem's ascent to (the second gate) between the kidneys. If the latter is blocked and the gem remains stationary, his companion should *pinch* the backbone there to help its ascent. However, if the practiser thinks of pushing it up, which is wrong, he will fail to raise it, for as soon as a thought stirs his heart, the second gate will close of itself. Hence the method of the *'five dragons upholding the holy one'* was devised to speed the gem's ascent.

Although the passage of the 'precious gem' is blocked and although neither stirring in the heart nor concentration of spirit can set it moving, the companion's *pinch* will warm and loosen the marrow in the second gate (to let it pass). In addition the practiser should *press* a finger on the mortal gate (at the root of the penis), and vitality in the precious gem will of itself thrust through the second gate (between the kidneys).

Therefore, the practiser should not concentrate on pushing the agent (or gem) to set it moving but wait for it to thrust of itself, and then gently guide it into the right channel. When it suddenly moves to thrust through the second gate the practiser should help the movement by *pressing* a finger on the mortal gate, looking up at the same time to draw it up. Then he should roll his eyes once quickly, acting like a *deer speedily drawing a cart uphill,* in order to raise the precious gem rapidly. In so doing he should support this ascent by *pressing* his tongue against the palate and *sucking* in a breath through the nose. Finally if he stretches the small of his back with a crack, the agent will of itself thrust into the second gate.

Now his companion should quickly *pinch* the backbone above the second gate (between the kidneys) and the 'precious gem' will gradually ascend to the third gate in the occiput. If the latter is blocked and the gem remains stationary there, his companion should *pinch* the back of the head to ease its ascent. For it cannot be moved by the practiser's thought and concentration but by itself because of the companion's *pinch* which warms and loosens the marrow in the third gate. The practiser by *pressing* a finger on the mortal gate, causes the gem to thrust into the occiput, but he should wait until it enters it before guiding it into the correct channel. When it suddenly thrusts of itself through the back of the head, the practiser should immediately look up to support its ascent. This is what we call the *'five dragons upholding the holy one'* in its ascent.

The practiser should now force his eyes up acting like *an ox drawing a cart uphill.* He should support this ascent by *pressing* the tongue on the palate and *sucking* in a breath through the nose. Finally if he stretches the small of his back with a crack, the gem will of itself thrust into the occiput.

Now his companion should quickly *pinch* the nape of his neck to warm and loosen the marrow there so that the gem can slowly enter the 'store house of the wind' (feng fu, a cavity in the back of the head), the medulla oblongata, the cerebellum and the vital cavity of nature-spirit in the centre of the cerebrum. When life-vitality meets nature-spirit they unite and stay in the same cavity; the practiser should use a clothes-peg to shut his nostrils, quickly close his eyes and roll them from left to right nine times, and then pause to gaze at the light of vitality that appears in that cavity. This exercise of rolling the eyes is to be done four times, making 9 x 4 or thirty-six turns, during which his eye should be rolled thus:

to lift up the positive yang.

After this, he should open his eyes and roll them from right to left, and then close them to gaze at the light of vitality.

This should be done four times, making 6 x 4 or twenty-four turns, during which the eyes should be rolled thus:

to lower the negative yin.

This rolling of the eyes will cause spirit and vitality to unite into one single gem which is called the prenatal true seed (hsien t'ien chen chung).

When he turns his eyes down, this true seed in the original cavity of spirit (tsu ch'iao between and behind the eyes) will descend from the forehead to seek an outlet through the nose, which is open, and if the latter is not shut by a clothes-peg, it will drain away by the nostrils, and all previous progress will be nullified. This is the danger of a fall from the upper magpie-bridge (shang ch'ueh ch'iao, the nasal duct).

Therefore, the practiser should provide himself with a wooden bun and a clothes-peg for use at this stage. If the true seed does not drain away by the nose and is stationary between the eyebrows, the practiser should remain thoughtless and motionless with his spirit frozen and look down while waiting for the true seed to move of itself. Suddenly it will thrust and the practiser should follow and guide it into the hsuan ying cavity (the mysterious bridle behind the heavenly pool above the mouth) and the throat where another peril should be anticipated. If he has not received instruction from a competent master he will spurt the true seed (out of his mouth) but if he has been instructed he will swallow it, and after passing down the throat it will reach the heart and the liver at the base of which is the chiang kung cavity (the solar plexus) where it mingles with the negative breath in the liver. With his eyes fixed on it, the true seed will reach the intestines in the middle of which is the channel of function (jen mo) and then slip into the lower tan t'ien cavity (under the navel) where it will remain stationary.

Thus after passing through the three gates in the backbone the true seed is now absorbed to achieve the alchemical goal.

Question You have said that the method of the '*five dragons upholding the holy one*' ensures the final breakthrough; will you please explain this in detail?

Answer Five is the number of the element of earth which stands for right thought, and *dragon* stands for prenatal spirit. Hence the '*five dragons upholding the holy one*' (wu lung p'eng sheng) which is the secret of the breakthrough by the macrocosmic alchemical agent.

Question I am still not very clear about the '*five dragons upholding the holy one*' and pray you to explain in detail.

Answer When the practiser gathers the macrocosmic alchemical agent for the final breakthrough, he should take advantage of the moment when all six sense organs shake, that is when the immortal seed vibrates, to sit firmly on the wooden bun in order to close his anus, and then the mortal gate (at the root of the penis) will shut of itself. He should also check that gate by pressing a finger on it. The right thought is symbolised by the element of earth whose number is *five*. Spirit is the *dragon*, which is the adept who is ready to sacrifice his body in his quest of immortality. When the precious gem vibrates to take its (transcendental) course, the practiser should relinquish his body, and this means its (apparent) death. For when he goes against the way of the world, he will achieve immortality. This reversal of the worldly way of life consists of holding up the mortal gate with a hand, backed by his right thought, so that the precious gem will soar up. Looking up to suck the gem up is *upholding* it. The *holy one* is the ascending precious gem.

Therefore, the method of '*five dragons upholding the holy one*' is only an analogy used by former patriarchs and masters who did not go into details. My masters Liao Jan and Liao K'ung have ordered me to explain it in detail so that all future students will benefit from it.

Question The gathering of the macrocosmic alchemical agent in seven days for the breakthrough also includes the four techniques of *sucking* (hsi), *pressing* (shih), *pinching* (ts'o) and *shutting* (pi). Will you please explain in detail?

Answer Sucking, pressing, pinching and *shutting* are the whole process of gathering the macrocosmic alchemical agent in seven days for the final breakthrough.

Sucking is drawing breath up the nostrils while looking up to help the true gem ascend. Both sucking and right thought support the upward look to ensure the ascent of the true gem.

Pressing is pressing the tongue against the palate. When the true seed ascends, it should be supported by the breath in the nasal duct and the upward look as well as the tongue pressing on the palate; at the same time the eyes should roll once from left to right. When the eyes are being rolled, the practiser should distinguish between the various strengths of the goat, deer and ox when drawing the cart uphill.

Pinching is done by the practiser's companion who should squeeze the channel of control (tu mo, in the spine). When the gem vibrates, the anus is blocked by the wooden bun and the mortal gate (at the root of the penis) is pressed by the practiser's own finger to stop the gem from slipping away by these two gates. The companion should now quickly pinch the base of the spine to warm and loosen the marrow there so that the gem thrusts into it with a crack. After this the companion should pinch the backbone between the kidneys, and then the back of the head until the gem has passed through the second and third gates and reached the brain.

Shutting is by means of the wooden bun that closes the anus, the clothes-peg that shuts the nasal duct and the finger that presses on the mortal gate (at the root of the penis). Thus these three gates are shut to stop the gem from slipping away.

Question After gathering the macrocosmic alchemical agent

and its ascent through the three gates (in the backbone) to the brain (ni wan) it will unite with the ni wan to become the true gem. Why then is the technique of ascent and descent still practised at this stage?

Answer This true gem is the *left-vitality* of the immortal seed which goes up through the three gates to the brain (ni wan) where it meets and unites with *nature-vitality* to become one whole which is the prenatal true seed of immortality.

The technique of positive ascent and negative descent is practised to sublimate *nature-vitality* which is negative and *lift-vitality* which is positive, unite both into one true seed and transform the latter into golden nectar which then goes down, but is not the saliva in the mouth. If the nostrils are not shut with a clothes-peg this nectar will drain away by it.

From the original cavity of spirit (between and behind the eyes) this golden nectar will pass through the hsuan ying cavity (above the mouth) to flow into the throat. When it goes down into the windpipe, if the practiser has not received instruction from a competent master, he will simply cough it up. Is it not a pity then that all previous progress is thus thrown away?

Hence the Scriptures say: 'Before the nectar goes down, the practiser should moisten the windpipe so that when the former descends it will be swallowed by the latter with a gulping noise. It will then enter the heart and reach the chiang kung cavity (solar plexus) under the liver where the (vital) breath there will invigorate it. It will then pass through the intestines and finally enter the lower tan t'ien (under the navel) where it will produce the true seed which will blossom and bear fruit.

Question You have said that the golden nectar will produce the true seed which will blossom and bear fruit in the cavity of vitality (under the navel). I am not clear about this; will you explain in detail?

Answer It is not easy to produce the true seed from the golden nectar. This seed will grow in the cavity of vitality (under the navel) into a yellow stem which will blossom and bear fruit. Its flower is the light of vitality which manifests in front of the practiser. This flower has both stamen and pistil which will unite to form a fruit. If the practiser does not know how to unite them the flower will be sterile and will not bear fruit, for it will be illusory. Its pistil is the light of vitality that comes from nature-vitality and its stamen is the golden light that arises from life-vitality. The union of both produces the (immortal) foetus which is the fruit.

14

FORMATION OF THE
IMMORTAL FOETUS

After his successful practice of the thirteen previous steps (Chapters 1 to 13) has achieved the breakthrough, the practiser should unite the two vitalities (of nature and life) to help spirit form the immortal foetus. Forgetfulness of (i.e. not thinking about) the circulation of the two vitalities (in the microcosmic orbit) will produce the foetal spirit which will return to the state of utter serenity which is true foetal breath.

Question Will you please explain all this in detail?

Answer After having gathered the macrocosmic alchemical agent and circulated it through the three gates of the backbone, all psychic centres (and channels) are cleared of obstructions so that the two vitalities (of nature and life) which have now developed fully, can move freely by themselves, ascending and descending endlessly; this is how the two vitalities help spirit produce the (immortal) foetus.

As time passes, they will circulate of themselves without the practiser being aware of it; this is how to produce the foetal spirit.

After a long time, while this mindless circulation continues, the practiser should concentrate his eyes on the lower tan t'ien centre (beneath the navel). Ten months later the circulation of the two vitalities (of nature and life) will become so subtle that only a feeble vibration is felt in the region of the navel which seems to be empty. One year later this vibration will cease completely. At this stage the practiser should not take salt when eating or drinking. Now only spirit remains, serene and radiant, which is true foetal breath. Breathing will (appear to) stop and all pulses to cease beating; the state of deep serenity (ta ting) is now achieved.

The foetal breath will remain still for a long time, and the heart, spirit and thought will start vibrating again causing the former to move like a louse; this is the spiritual foetus which, after remaining inert in the lower tan t'ien centre (under the navel) for about two years since the breakthrough, now begins to breathe. At this stage the practiser should lift this true foetal breath to the chung kung, also called chiang kung, centre which is (the solar plexus) at the base of the liver, by means of the threefold continual ascension method (san ch'ien fa)[1] After reaching the chung kung centre (solar plexus), the spiritual foetus will be nurtured by the foetal breath.

The lower tan t'ien under the navel is where the generative force is sublimated into vitality; the middle tan t'ien (solar plexus) is where vitality is sublimated into spirit; and the upper tan t'ien in the brain (ni wan) is where spirit is sublimated for its flight into space.

---

[1]San ch'ien fa or threefold continual ascension method means the three essentials, i.e. the generative force, vitality and spirit united into a bright moonlight which rises from the lower to the middle and then the upper tan t'ien before the practiser sees falling snow and dancing flowers in front of him.

圖 胎 道

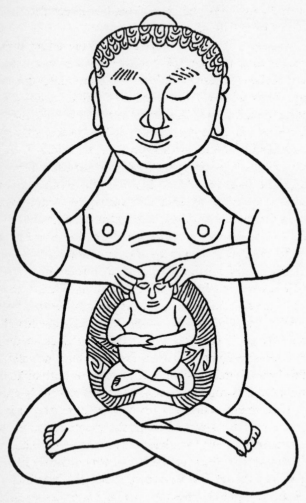

Figure 10 The immortal foetus

When the spiritual foetus takes shape, the practiser should employ the threefold continual ascension method which uses thoughtlessness in the first and breathlessness in the second stages (i.e. he should neither direct the process mentally nor regulate his breathing).

The stage of foetal breathlessness is achieved by 'uniting' the eyes (by drawing the pupils together in a squint) to concentrate on the foetal vitality in the lower tan t'ien (under the navel) to cause the foetal breath to ascend slowly, little by little, to the middle tan t'ien (or the solar plexus). This means that the spirit which has been in (the cavity of) vitality (i.e. the lower tan t'ien) for some time now moves to ascend to the middle tan t'ien where vitality will envelop the foetal spirit which will be dull, confused and indistinct, like a foetus in the mother's womb. This is the stage of breathlessness. When spirit is enveloped by vitality in the middle tan t'ien, it is called the immortal foetus (tao t'ai). That this foetus is forming is revealed by foetal vitality manifesting before the practiser's eyes as the light of vitality.

It is very difficult for the practiser to refrain from using this manifestating vitality (which is tempting). He has to bury the heart (the seat of the fire of passion) in order to resurrect (essential) nature; he should not allow himself to be held back by house work, or entangled in worldly activities so that all mundane things can be kept away for ever. Then he will know only this light of vitality beyond which there is nothing to concern him; this is complete relinquishment of all earthly attachments. If there still remains a trace of negative breath in the body, demonic states will develop; the practiser should then employ the method for banishing demons (see opposite);

The above are the four stages of serenity, the sequence of which is: (a) thoughtlessness (nien chu), (b) breathlessness (hsi chu), (c) pulselessness (mo chu) and (d) extinction (unmindfulness) of worldly existence (mich chin).

Question You have said that when the foetal breath ascends to the middle tan t'ien (in the solar plexus), it will be enveloped by the prenatal vitality there and will become the immortal foetus; and that foetal vitality manifests before the practiser's eyes, as the light of vitality. How then can worldly things and demonic visions manifest in that light of vitality?

Answer When the immortal foetus is nurtured in the middle tan t'ien, the heart is like a lotus leaf which cannot be wetted by water; so the practiser (who has achieved this stage) is at ease, free, comfortable and unconcerned about anything. When the immortal foetus is fully developed, its vitality will manifest before his eyes. Spirit which is now wholly positive can develop vitality with its six transcendental powers and achieves: 1, the stoppage of all drain (of generative and vital forces); 2, divine sight; 3, divine hearing; 4, knowledge of past lives; 5, understanding of other minds; and 6, the divine mirror.

Previously when the student began his practice, he had succeeded in stopping the drain of generative force; it is only now that he realises the other five spiritual powers which enable him (a) to see things in heaven, (b) to hear celestial sounds and voices, (c) to know all causes sown in past lives, and (d) to read the minds of others and predict the future, except for (e) the divine mirror which will remain tied to consciousness if he does not know how to free his heart (the seat of the fire of passion) from worldly attachments. If he gives rise to the thought of seeking immortality to delight in it, the demon will seize the occasion to enter his heart. His discrimination and likes and dislikes will cause demonic states to manifest thereby destroying all his previous progress.

When the student feels that consciousness interferes with his practice he should immediately call on a learned master who will teach him the method of overcoming the demons by circulating his consciousness through the four cardinal points A, D, G and J (of the microcosmic orbit). The demons will vanish as soon as the negative breath is transmuted into positive vitality. This is the death of consciousness leading to the resurrection of (essential) nature. Hence the divine mirror which is achieved only after positive fire has transmuted the demons into prenatal (divine) spirit.

Question When the immortal foetus which has been sufficiently nurtured by prenatal vitality in the chung kung centre (the solar plexus) is being pushed up to the upper tan t'ien in the brain (ni wan) there may or may not be a foretelling sign. If there is not, when should the foetus be pushed up?

Answer There is always a foretelling sign. Without one how can the practiser know when the moment is ripe to push up the immortal foetus to the brain (ni wan)? This sign is the golden light appearing in the bright moonlight that manifests before the practiser's eyes; this is when the foetus should be pushed up. The practiser should immediately drive the golden light into his (essential) nature, and unite negative and positive spirits to sustain it. The positive spirit is still weak and is like a baby; this is why a method called 'giving suck' should be used to nurture it. According to this method that which is void (formless) is not really empty for there is in it a golden light; hence it is not void. Simultaneously the original cavity of spirit (tsu ch'iao between and behind the eyes) will emit bright moonlight, and when the two lights unite, the positive spirit which is serene and radiant in the upper tan t'ien (in the brain or ni wan) will mingle with them to become a vast voidness. This is how to nurture and preserve the whole body (of positive spirit) which is the chief aim of the method of 'giving suck' to the spiritual foetus. When the practiser achieves this, he will be aware of the egress of spirit from the body. This is the ascent of the immortal foetus to the upper tan t'ien in the brain (or ni wan).

By threefold continual ascension is meant the union of generative force, vitality and spirit into one whole which will be sublimated into bright moonlight. It is only after flying snow and falling heavenly flowers have been seen that spirit emerges from the foetus to become immortal.

Question You said that the threefold ascension is from the lower, middle and upper tan t'ien centres and that the lower centre (under the navel) is where the generative force is transmuted into the immortal or true seed, the middle tan t'ien (solar plexus) is where vitality is transmuted into the immortal foetus, and the upper tan t'ien in the brain (or ni wan) is where spirit is sublimated so that it can come out of the foetus. I am not very clear about the generative force which can become the immortal seed and the immortal foetus and can emerge from the upper tan t'ien (in the brain or ni wan) to become immortal. Will you please explain all this in detail?

Answer You know that sexual intercourse produces offspring. When the male spermatozoon enters the female ovum which has not yet been stirred, the woman's blood will surround the semen and the offspring will be a girl who is negative externally and positive internally. When the female ovum is stirred before the male spermatozoon enters it, the man's sperm will surround the woman's blood and the issue will be a boy who is positive externally and negative internally.

According to our Taoist teaching, in the human body the union of spirit with vitality begets the immortal seed which comes from the sublimation of semen, for when spirit and vitality unite in the lower tan t'ien (under the navel) they collect all spermatozoa and transform them into immortal seed. When the latter is sufficiently nurtured and matures it radiates. Spirit and vitality will then become inseparable like iron and a loadstone.

This achievement is final and the practiser will feel secure and independent. Consciousness will gradually vanish while essential nature will develop slowly. Perverse thoughts will cease to arise giving way to one right thought. The union of spirit and vitality means the death of consciousness and the resurrection of essential nature. Heart and thought which are now neither within nor without become a mass of serenity which will remain still for a long time before vibrating again.

This is vibration of the true seed which will soar up to the chung kung centre, also called chiang kung (or solar plexus) where it will stay. This centre is where vitality and (vital) breath unite to produce prenatal true vitality, which contributes to the formation of the immortal foetus.

This immortal foetus is formed by the union of two prenatal vitalities: prenatal true nature-vitality in (essential) nature whose light is like moonlight and prenatal true life-vitality in (eternal) life whose light is golden.

When this stage is reached the practiser should not dwell in the inactive (wu wei) state but should direct the (active) inner (vital) breath to reach and enter the prenatal true vitality in order to invigorate and help it form and nurture the immortal foetus.

The practiser should now use the vitality in his heart to still the inner breath for if (vital) breath is not regulated the immortal foetus cannot develop fully. He should concentrate on spirit forgetting all about the foetus which is within his spirit; this is called 'returning a myriad things to one whole'.

This one true vitality is the positive vitality of (essential) nature which will unite with the negative vitality of (eternal) life to become that one basic vitality which reveals the complete formation of the immortal foetus. The latter should be quickly lifted to the ni wan or brain. This is ascent to the upper tan t'ien where the union of (positive) with (negative) spirit and their return to the brain will produce one uniform prenatal positive spirit.

The union of (positive) with (negative) spirit is achieved by uniting (or drawing together in a squint) the pupil of the left eye which stands for positive spirit with that of the right one which stands for negative spirit for concentration on the upper tan t'ien centre (in the brain). At this stage breath will not (be felt to) enter or leave (the body), the serenity experienced is full of bliss, and the six senses are blotted out to reveal one essential nature which is perfect and radiant with the shining and pervading light of vitality. When this light manifests, there will be neither day nor night; this shining and pervading brightness will give the practiser great comfort and he will acquire all six supernatural powers. This is the highest attainment.

As time passes, he will discover many (unusual) things; he should not use this vitality but should hold on to the ni wan centre in order not to be disturbed by consciousness. This is what is usually called the extinction (of worldly things) which is full of bliss. This extinction is neither death nor annihilation but confirms the fullness and maturity of the immortal foetus which is like a bright sun in mid-heaven.

This is absolute voidness which is not empty. When snow appears to dance in space while flowers fall in disorder from the sky, this is the time for (the spirit) to come out of the foetus. If (the spirit) does not emerge at this stage it is called *'keeping vigil over a dead body'*.

Question You have spoken of dancing snow and falling flowers; where and why do flowers fall from the sky?

Answer When (positive) unites with (negative) spirit to produce one uniform prenatal spirit, the latter derives from the
union of nature and life vitalities as shown in the following
diagram:

Only when this foetus has been nurtured by vitality, and

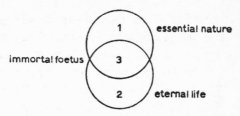

is full and mature can flowers be seen falling from the sky
before the eyes, which shows the time is ripe for leaving the
foetus which should be done immediately. Dancing snow
reveals the full development of the immortal foetus.

The patriarch Hua Yang commenting on the Hui Ming
Ching said: 'This is the time to come out of serenity. If the
practiser does not leave this state he will get bogged down in
the spiritual body, will be tied up by serenity and will not
achieve the transcendental powers which enable him to appear
in myriad transformation bodies. When snow and flowers are
seen, spirit should leave the mortal body *stirred by the thought*
of entering the great emptiness.[2] He who has not received
instruction from a competent master does not know this
method.'

Question The Hui Ming Ching says: 'He who has not received
instruction from a competent master does not know how to *stir
the thought* of entering the great emptiness.' It does not teach
the method of leaving the foetus; will you please instruct me?

---

[2]*Stirred by a thought* (tung nien) is a Taoist idiom which means the mind set
solely on entering the great emptiness, the aim of alchemy.

Answer You should lift the spiritual light to the brain (ni wan) which will emit the light of vitality within which flying snow and dancing flowers will be seen. This is the absolute void taking shape. Although there seems to be activity this in fact is wu wei (non-activity) and although a shape seems to form this in reality is the sublimation of spirit; this is sublimation both within and without.

An ancient immortal said: 'Shape is formed by Tao (immortality) and life is made eternal through alchemy which consists of borrowing boundless prenatal vitality to continue (the existence of) limited bodily form; in other words this boundless prenatal vitality which is the true essence of the positive and negative principles between heaven and earth, is used to create the immortal foetus which now has shape'. This is the union of (positive) and (negative) spirits which produces the immortal foetus. The latter derives from the union of the spiritual father and mother in the (practiser's) body; in other words the union of the true positive and negative principles. The postnatal (human) foetus created by the sexual intercourse of the father and mother takes ten months to become a baby, the product of his parents' vital forces. Likewise the immortal foetus which comes from the union of positive and negative vitalities in the practiser's own body also takes ten months to complete.

When flowers are seen falling in disorder from the sky, the practiser should use the method of *stirring a thought* to jump into the great emptiness, and he will emerge from the immortal foetus.

When the lights of (essential) nature and (eternal) life unite the foetus will take the form of the (practiser's) self which is created by the spiritual father and mother, that is by the positive and negative vitalities in his own body. In other words this is the union of his positive and negative spirits which creates his true spirit which can transform his bodily self into vapour which then gathers to take shape. This is prenatal vitality in the pre-natal state which in fact is wholly positive vitality, or *positive spirit* created by the five kinds of eyes (see below) and six transcendental powers, which is visible to others, can speak to them, can pick up objects and has the same features as his own body.

The *negative spirit* visible to the practiser when he closes his eyes, is created by (the first) five transcendental powers and is the negative spiritual breath which can see others but is invisible to them, cannot speak to them and cannot pick up objects and is, therefore, mortal in the end whereas positive spirit enjoys eternal life and is beyond birth and death.

If the heavenly gate (miao men or aperture of Brahma at the top of the head) is not open, the positive spirit will not come out (of the body) and the practiser will remain a stupid man; this is because he has not met a competent master. I, therefore, urge all students to call on learned masters for verbal instruction on the method of *stirring the thought* to open the heavenly gate in order to leap into the great emptiness. All my disciples know this method; hence I advise all practisers to call on them for verbal instructions.

Question What are the five kinds of eye?

Answer They are the heavenly, earthly, spiritual, human and ghostly eyes. The heavenly eye sees all things in the thirty-three heavens; the earthly eye sees the eighteen hells; the spiritual eye, or eye of vitality, sees both past and future events in the world; the human eye sees things happening before birth and death; and the ghostly eye sees through the mountains, earth and metal.

15

THE EGRESS

We have dealt with the creation of the positive and negative spirits as taught by competent masters. The positive spirit is visible to men whereas the negative spirit (is invisible to them but) can see them. When the practiser reaches this stage, if he has not received authentic instruction he will only produce the negative spirit and will become a seer of the plane of ghosts and spirits. By the creation of positive spirit is meant the opening of the heavenly gate (miao men at the top of the head). If the latter is shut the negative spirit will manifest. The opening of the miao men ensures the realisation of the six supernatural powers, the permanence of radiant heart-nature and the bright light of vitality.

The previous fourteenth step (Chapter 14) taught the stages of ascension (of the immortal foetus) and dealt with the method of nurturing it with generative force, vitality and spirit. It consists of developing the voidness which is even more void and the emptiness which is even more empty so that (essential) nature is like empty space and free from attachment thereto; hence it is called absolute voidness. If there is clinging to the concept of empty space it will hinder the realisation of absolute voidness. This absolute voidness will then be natural without

圖 胎 出

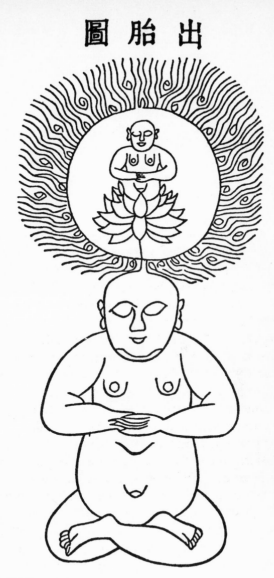

Figure 11 The egress

(even) the idea of existence. This is the right method of uniting inmost (essential) nature with inmost (eternal) life, and has nothing to do with the closing of one's eyes to sit motionless in meditation.

The serenity of the foetus depends solely on the practiser's unflinching faith; and during the ten months of its formation his mind should be set uniquely on it. (At this stage) neither the mouth nor the heart (i.e. neither words nor thoughts) are directed to the foetus whose serenity results from stopping the thinking process, and regulating the breath which brings about its full development and maturity.

When the practiser sees flying snow and falling flowers, he should, in order to leave the immortal foetus, hasten to give rise to the thought of leaping into the great emptiness, which will open the heavenly gate (miao men) of the sun and the moon (i.e. the two eyes) which he, now free from feelings and passions, and in accord with (essential) nature, should roll so that the two lights meet. This is the method of coming out of the foetus which the ancients did not lightly disclose for it should not be revealed to those who have not received instruction from competent masters.

Question Will you please explain in detail the method of realising this egress?

Answer This method was only verbally transmitted from masters to disciples and was not lightly revealed in books, but I was ordered to make it available to all serious practisers of alchemy. So I deal with it here.

In reality there was a method of coming out of the immortal foetus to appear in (countless) transformation bodies, but it is not easy to obtain it now. Formerly there was an adept called Lan Yang Su who had fully developed his immortal foetus and had seen flowers falling in disorder from the sky, but since he had not received instruction from competent masters, he failed to achieve the egress; so he was as ignorant as any worldly man in spite of (the possibility of attaining) eternal life lasting as long as heaven and earth. Later the patriarch Liu Hai Shan sent him the following poem:

> Though realisation comes from manifesting the divine
> Never let its (great) attractiveness handicap your body.
> Just follow the immortal Wu's method of liberation
> And when the foetus is mature you'll leap over the
> mundane.

After receiving the poem Lan Yang Su clapped his hands joyfully and immediately emerged from the foetus. This was the patriarch Wu's teaching.

The patriarch Liu Hua Yang said: 'When snow and flowers are seen falling and the time has come to leave the human body, give rise to the thought of leaving and direct it towards the great emptiness. He who has not met a competent master does not know this teaching.'

My masters Liao Jen and Liao K'ung said: 'Gather the five vitalities and return them to the source (the upper tan t'ien in the brain) where the union of (positive and negative) vitalities will produce the immortal foetus.'

My elder brother Kuei I Tsu said: 'When the three essences (i.e. the generative force, vitality and spirit) gather in the brain, the moonlight shines brighter; when the five (vital) breaths soar up to the head, the golden light will appear; and when the two (positive and negative) vitalities unite and return to the essential body, the spiritual self will appear in its centre.'

All the above teachings deal with egress from the foetus; although they differ in wording the underlying doctrine is the same. When the foetus is fully developed, snow and flowers are seen falling in disorder; this is visible to the (practiser's) eyes. When the five (vital) breaths in the heart, liver, stomach, lungs and kidneys gather in the head, spirit will break through the original cavity of spirit (between and behind the eyes) to ascend to the heavenly gate (miao men) from which it will leap into the great emptiness. The teaching formulates the gathering of *five* (vital) breaths, the crowding together of *four* cardinal points (A.G.D.J.) into the centre (chung kung or the solar plexus), the intermingling of *three* (components, i.e. the generative force, vitality and spirit) and the union of *two* (positive and negative) spirits into one whole.

According to the underlying doctrine, when the body is unstirred, the generative force is stabilised and the element of water moves to the head; when the heart is not stirred, the breath consolidates and the element of fire moves to the head; when (essential) nature is serene the incorporeal soul will be hidden and the element of wood moves to the head; when passions cease, the corporeal soul is subdued and the element of metal moves to the head; when these four elements (water, fire, wood and metal) are in harmony, the intellect is stable and the element of earth moves to the head. Thus all five (vital) breaths converge in the head as follows:

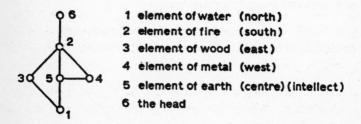

1 element of water (north)
2 element of fire (south)
3 element of wood (east)
4 element of metal (west)
5 element of earth (centre) (intellect)
6 the head

Figure 12 The five elements

When the five (vital) breaths converge in the head, the golden light appears and unites with the light of vitality which has manifested after the intermingling of the three essential compounds (i.e. the generative force, vitality and spirit). This is the union of the true positive and negative principles from which the immortal foetus emerges to take shape.

No foetus can be produced in a sterile male body, for to do so there must be a creative cause that drives (vital) breath into the cavity of vitality (the lower tan t'ien centre under the navel) to form a (spiritual) foetus there. After its formation, the practiser should gather the five (vital) breaths and drive them up to the head in order to force open the original cavity of spirit (tsu ch'iao between and behind the eyes). When the heavenly gate (miao men at the top of the head) opens, the two lights which have gathered in the original cavity of spirit will emerge to develop into a mass of golden light the size of a large wheel within which positive spirit (i.e. the immortal man) sits upright while the red light of his negative breath changes into a demon who will use all tricks to tempt him. If the heart (mind) allows itself to be attracted by what it sees and hears, the positive spirit will vanish giving way to the demon who will cause the practiser to transmigrate through the six realms of existence; thus all progress so far achieved will be thrown away. All this comes from wrong practice and lack of determination to put an end to mortality.

Question Will you please teach me how to remove this demonic hindrance in order to acquire a true undying body; is this body everlasting on earth?

Answer It is indispensable to hold on to the golden light unflinchingly. When encountering the demon you should practise the seventh step (Chapter 7) to unite the generative force, vitality and spirit in order to transform this demon into positive breath which will sustain the positive spirit and wipe out all demonic states.

To deal with the golden light that shrinks, the practiser should suck it in while rolling his eyes to drive it into the sea of (essential) nature (in the heart)[1] which will unite with it. After a serenity lasting for seven days, this light will shine and the negative principle will change into true spirit which will manifest in front of the practiser, with its features identical with his; this is the undying self.

When spirit manifests for the first time it should only be allowed to leave the physical body in fine weather and it should be well looked after, like a baby just born. Its egress should on no account take place when there is thick fog, heavy rain, gale, lightning and thunder.

When for the first time positive spirit comes out it should (be made to) return to the body at once. During the first three months it should be pulled out once a week. After this it will gradually develop perception and knowledge and is very sensitive to fear and awe which should be avoided at all costs.

Its egress and return to the body should be orderly and at regular intervals. Each coming out should be immediately followed by re-entry until the practiser is familiar with the exercise. It should take place in the day but never at night.

After six months positive spirit can be let out once every three days; and after a year once a day. During these exercises it should always be kept close to the body and not allowed to stray. In the case of fright and awe it should be quickly returned to the body. These instructions should be carried out carefully.

---

[1] The heart (the house of fire) is the seat of essential nature which manifests through the two eyes. When the heart is serene it reveals essential nature and when eternal life is mature the spiritual light appears.

After two years of exercise the egress can take place either in the day or at night and the number of times can be increased gradually. The positive spirit can now leave the body to wander inside or outside the grotto (place of meditation) and then return to the body to suck.[2]

After three years of exercise the practiser can send the positive spirit to distant places. If it meets men and animals it should return swiftly to the body. From now on it can cover a distance of half a mile or a mile and return quickly.

To sum up the positive principle should at the beginning of the exercise return to the body as soon as it is out of it until it is familiar with the practice. In short it should stay in the body much longer than outside it. After the practice has been successful for three years, the positive principle becomes an (earth-bound) immortal (shen hsien). Now is the time for a course of training which will enable this immortal to dwell in the state of serenity for nine years in order to return to the great emptiness thereby transforming his physical body into that of a golden immortal (chin hsien).

My master Liao K'ung said: 'When spirit soars up to the top of the head after breaking through its original cavity (between and behind the eyes), do not give rise to fear and awe; be bold and concentrate on the sole thought of getting out through the heavenly gate (in the top of the skull). Then close your eyes, turn them down and lift them gently as if to jump up; you will feel as if coming out of a dream and will see another body beside your own.' When positive spirit leaves the body it will stop about three to four feet away. If you see and hear something, do not let your heart (the seat of nature) be drawn to it, and pay no attention to visions of parents, relatives, friends, wife and children, or to other states; do not

[2] *Suck* is a Taoist term which means drawing nourishment from the body.

recognise them and avoid being influenced by them; do not cling to anything but stay unperturbed, cutting off all feelings and passions, with only the single thought of dwelling in the state of serenity while refusing to see and hear anything.

Shortly after dwelling in this serenity a golden light will emerge from the body like a large wheel, manifesting in front of the practiser who should drive the light of his spiritual nature in front of it, and imagine that the golden light shrinks into a small circle about one inch in diameter, like a gold coin. He should then roll his eyes to collect and suck (the golden light) into his spiritual nature which will enter the original cavity of spirit (tsu ch'iao, between and behind the eyes). After this he should practise the 'obliterating' meditation[3] in order to return to the state of stable serenity.

An ancient said: 'The golden light is a wonderful drug which changes form into nothingness; on no account should it be missed.' For if it scatters at this stage it will never return. Although some people like to preserve form, the latter cannot evaporate (in the absence of the golden light).

The master Liao Jen said: 'When the positive spirit leaves the body for the first time, the student should, after achieving complete serenity, practise the method of directing the five vitalities (to the head) and of giving rise to the single thought of stepping into the great emptiness in order to transform spirit into a golden light the size of a great wheel which should then unite with the light of his spiritual nature into one single light in the centre of which (the form of his) positive spirit sits upright.' At the same time the negative breath in that light will turn into a demon who will use all attractive states to entice the positive spirit. If the practiser allows himself to be tempted by what he sees and hears, the positive spirit will vanish and not

---

[3]Lit. 'extinguishing' meditation which will wipe away all traces of the worldly.

return, thereby causing him to enter demonic states and transmigrate through the six mortal realms of existence. People wrongly regard this as leaving the world while sitting in meditation and as achieving the mediocre fruit (attainment). If the practiser so fails all his previous progress will be thrown away. Is it not a pity? This failure is caused by wrong training and want of determination to put an end to mortality.

The remedying method consists of holding on to the golden light while dwelling in serenity with unflinching determination to banish the demon. Then all demonic states will vanish and the practiser should shrink the golden light, roll his eyes to suck it into his spiritual body, and return the latter to the original cavity of spirit (tsu ch'iao between and behind the eyes). After a long while the golden light will emerge again to transform the negative demon into positive spirit which will manifest in front of him. Only when the positive spirit appears with features identical to his can it be prevented from fleeing away.

The master Liu Ming Jui said: 'When the immortal foetus first comes out of the original cavity of spirit (tsu ch'iao) the practiser should guard against outside demonic disturbances, and should never speak to those apparitions that greet him but should hold on to the right thought (concentration). Spirit should return to the body as soon as it is out of it and should not go to distant places. The golden light the size of a large wheel that manifests two to three feet from his body belongs to him and should be sucked back into the body; it is a wonderful drug that will sublimate his body and return it to nothingness.

'When it emerges for the first time, it should not cling to anything outside; the practiser should drive his spiritual body in front of the golden light to absorb it, and draw the former into his physical body which will imbibe the light which will transform it into vapour. If he fails to get hold of the golden light his body will not evaporate.'

The master Liu Ch'uan Yang said: 'When positive spirit comes out of the original cavity of spirit and fails to return to the body, this is due to wrong training. Therefore, when the positive spirit goes out, it is most important to hold on to the golden light unflinchingly; then all demons will disappear. The positive spirit should not be allowed to go out carelessly but should be reabsorbed as soon as it has left, for once outside it may detest the filthy body and refuse to return to its unclean abode. It should be kept close to the body and returned to it until the practiser is familiar with the exercise.

'When it re-enters the brain (or ni wan) the body will feel hot as fire, and the golden light will radiate through all pores. If the practiser gives way to fright or delights in this light he will slip into the way of the demon and will fail in his training.

'To sum up the practiser should hold on to his dogged determination to achieve the aim of alchemy and be adamantine to all passions including pleasure, anger, sorrow and joy.'

The old master P'eng Mou Ch'ang said: 'When the positive spirit comes out for the first time, it is still very weak. If the light of vitality is to congeal and stop scattering away, it should be well nurtured so that it will gain in strength and become boundless. When the gold light manifests it should merge in the light of vitality; this is the union of true negative and positive lights into a single one with the holy foetus in the centre. This (spiritual body which has come out of the) holy foetus should be sucked back at once, which means subjecting it to the exercise of going out and returning. At the start it is inclined to waver and should be turned back to be controlled during the exercise so that it becomes stable. Hence the saying: "It should be stilled again and again" so that it grows and develops naturally.'

The master Liu Hua Yang said: 'I have read the stories of ancient immortals who were all liberated after undergoing the same training.' Students of coming generations reading this book will know the secrets of alchemy. There is no need for them to climb high mountains and cross streams and rivers to seek instructions from masters. If they are provided with the means (money) and have (helping) companions with them and practise seriously they will leap over the worldly to the saintly realms.

My brother Chao K'uei I said: 'Drive the positive spirit into the upper tan t'ien (in the brain or ni wan) which is under the heavenly gate (miao men at the top of the head) and look inward to produce divine fire there. With the fire of positive spirit in the head, the practiser should concentrate on it in silence so that the fire above will descend and the fire below will soar up; and that the five vitalities will converge in the head and break through the cavity of spirit (between and behind the eyes) to reach the source (of the nervous system, pai hui) from which the positive spirit will manifest. The brain will then be like a pond full of golden nectar with silvery ripples.

'After the five vitalities have thrust up into the top of the head like thunder, and forced open the inner heavenly palace (tzu fu, another name for the tzu ch'iao in the centre of the brain) a boundless red light will suddenly emerge, thundering at the original cavity of spirit (tsu ch'iao) to expose the practiser's self who is the positive spirit which should then be returned to the body. This exercise of egress once a week should continue for a period of three years at the end of which the positive spirit will have developed fully. At this stage the adept should practise its return to nothingness. I realised this after I had trained for over forty years.'

All the above methods were taught by my masters personally and although the wording differs the underlying principle is the same throughout. I took notes of what they told me so that future practisers can be clear about the training.

Question The above teachings on the egress from the foetus are clear but I am afraid that those who have not met competent masters will read your book with difficulty. Will you please explain the method in every day language so that those who have not met masters can understand it easily?

Answer The method consists of closing the eyes while sitting in meditation to drive the light of (essential) nature in front of the practiser who should 'unite' his eyes (by drawing the pupils together) so that a bright light like that of the moon appears in the centre (between the eyes). A long while later he will see snow and flowers falling in disorder in this moonlight, and should immediately give rise to the thought of leaping into the great emptiness.

This is the method of uniting the five vitalities in the heart, spleen, lungs, liver and kidneys into a single vitality which will then rise from the base of the spine and pass through the second gate (between the kidneys) and the back of the head to reach the brain (ni wan) and thrust through the original cavity of spirit (tsu ch'iao between and behind the eyes) to knock at the source of the nervous system (pai hui).

The practiser should look up quickly in order to force open the heavenly gate (at the top of the skull); this consists of opening the eyes to look up (and so give a) thrust to burst open the gate with the combined force of the heart, intellect and thought.

If the five vitalities are full a golden light will soar up to unite with the light of (essential) nature to become a single light which is the union of the radiant vitality of the positive principle (yang) in the head and the bright light of the negative principle (yin) in the abdomen into one single light which will result in the egress from the immortal foetus. The practiser should then lower his eyes slowly to look down before closing them with the combined force of his heart and intellect as if to make a jump. He will then feel as if waking from a dream to see another body beside his own.

This is the method of drawing the positive spirit out (of the foetus). If the practiser does not give rise to the thought of flying into space and fails to converge the five vitalities in the head) the spirit will not leave. Below is a diagram showing the five vitalities converging to the head before the egress of positive spirit.

The five vitalities unite into a single one which will rise from the base of the spine to the head to break through the original cavity of spirit before reaching the top of the head

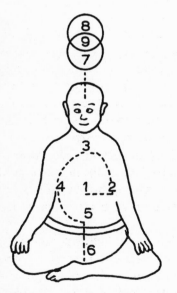

1 Vitality in the heart
2 Vitality in the spleen
3 Vitality in the lungs
4 Vitality in the liver
5 Vitality in the kidneys
6 Descent to the base of the spine before rising in the backbone to the head
7 The negative principle
8 The positive principle
9 Egress from the foetus

Figure 13 The five vitalities converging to the head.

where the golden light of the true negative principle meets the moonlight of the true positive principle in order to beget the immortal foetus in the centre (where both lights meet). The practiser should now lower his eyes to look down so that his spiritual body will manifest with his physical body at its side. His spiritual body is similar in features to his physical body but traces of negative vitality in the former will cause demonic hindrance by all sorts of states to tempt the positive spirit. The practiser should now hold on to the right concentration and quickly roll his eye once from cardinal point A to D, G and J (see *figure 5* on page 72) while concentrating on the demonic light to suck it into his body in order to transmute it into positive light. As time passes this demonic light will be purified and transformed into the light of positive spirit which will sustain the foetus in its full development. After this the practiser should continue his still meditation in order to return the positive spirit to nothingness.

16

APPEARING IN SPACE

My master Liao K'ung said: 'The return to nothing-ness is achieved in the final stage of training in which the practiser, while maintaining serenity of heart, lets the all-embracing positive spirit leave his bodily form to appear in the world and to perform its work of salvation such as alleviating human sufferings, curing the sick, etc. and then re-enter its original cavity (tsu ch'iao, between and behind the eyes) in order to be preserved in the ocean of (essential) nature. It should not be allowed again to leave the body, which now should be closed and further sublimated in order to enter the spiritual body which comprises (essential) nature and (eternal) life in their prenatal condition. The physical body is then further sublimated so that it is neither existing nor non-existent, neither form nor void, neither within nor without, neither coming nor going, and neither beginning nor ending. This is done with the same care that a dragon nurtures its pearl while remaining hidden and motionless, and because of which a sitting hen refuses to leave her eggs; this condition of quiet and stillness should be held until it reaches its highest degree.'

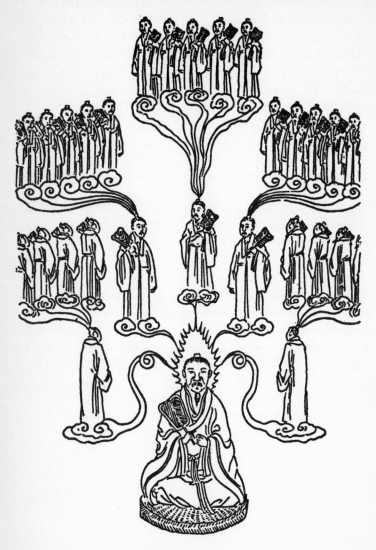

Figure 14 Countless transformation bodies appearing in space

All previous achievements such as appearing in countless transformation bodies riding on dragons and storks,[1] walking on the sun and playing with the moon, as well as thousands of transmutations should now be gathered in the original cavity of spirit (between and behind the eyes) in order to be reduced to the state of complete stillness and extinction. This is called the condition of a hibernating dragon. It leads to the complete extinction (of all phenomena) which should be carefully maintained in order to prevent positive spirit from going out (leaving the body), so that it can be further sublimated to reach its highest degree. This continual sublimation will result in deeper concealment of the spiritual fire in the light of vitality so that the positive spirit will be kept in its original cavity (tsu ch'iao). As time passes while dwelling in utter serenity, the true fire of positive spirit will develop fully and radiate inside and outside its cavity to become all-embracing, shining on heaven, earth and myriad things which will appear within its light.

The training should continue no matter how long it takes until the four elements[2] (that make the body) scatter, and space pulverises leaving no traces behind; this is the golden immortal stage of the indestructible diamond-body. This is the ultimate achievement of the training which now comes to an end.

---

[1] Dragon and stork are emblems of longevity.
[2] Body, breath, corporeal and incorporeal souls. See also note 3 on page 36.

GLOSSARY

Alchemical agents, The three:

1 The *microcosmic outer* alchemical agent is produced by *outer* fresh air breathed in and out to restore the generative force which has drained away in order to purify and transmute it into vitality.

2 The *microcosmic inner* alchemical agent is produced by the *inner* vital breath in the body which transmutes vitality into spirit.

3 The *macrocosmic* alchemical agent is gathered to break through the original cavity of spirit in the brain for the mortal man to become immortal, i.e. for the integration of microcosm into macrocosm.

Alchemical agent, The three components of the: The generative force, vitality and spirit.

Alchemical process, The four phases of: Move (hsin), stay (chu), re-start (chi) and stop (chih). The element of fire in the generative force, vitality and spirit *moves* from A to D (for cleansing) and then to G where it *stays* for a while and is called the ascending positive fire; and subsequently *re-starts* from G to J (for purification) and then *stops* at A (see *figure 2*) and is called the descending negative fire.

Alchemy, Taoist: An ancient science which teaches the stopping of the flow of the generative force inherent in every man so that instead of being discharged to procreate offspring or to waste away, it is retained in the body for purification and transmutation into positive vitality to restore original spirit which existed before the world came into being and so that it can return to its primal immortal state.

All-pervading one, The: See I kuan

Ambrosia (kan lu): The sublimation of the generative force, vitality and spirit in the brain produces the ambrosia which, flowing in the mouth, becomes a liquid (saliva) which, when swallowed, makes sounds in the abdomen. This ambrosia produces and nurtures the immortal seed in the lower tan t'ien whence it radiates, lighting up the heart to reveal the formation of the immortal seed. See Kan lu and Sweet dew.

Ascent and descent of inner fire in the microcosmic orbit: When breathing in, the heart, spirit and thought should rise together in the channel of control from the cardinal point A at the base of the penis to the cardinal point G on the top of the head, and when breathing out, the heart, spirit and thought should together go down in the channel of function from the cardinal point G to A (see *figure 2)*. The ascent is positive and the descent is negative.

Audible vibration at the back of the head: It reveals the strength of fire in the generative force, vitality and spirit. It differs from the wrong type of fire which causes buzzing in the ear.

Bellows (t'o yo): The mechanism of ventilation in the body caused by in and out breathing to kindle the psychic fire in the lower abdomen like a bellows used for blowing fire.

Blazing fire in the lower tan t'ien: It shows the fullness of the generative force and vitality from which it arises.

Body, Essential (fa shen): Spiritual body of an immortal.

Breath, Vital: Breath of life which keeps the heart, stomach, liver, lungs and lower abdomen functioning, and without which the body perishes. When the white and golden lights unite, concentration in the head of these five vital breaths produces the macrocosmic alchemical agent which should be gathered for the final breakthrough thereby causing the practiser to leap over the worldly to the saintly state, and so leaving the state of serenity to appear in countless transformation bodies in the macrocosm.

Breathing, Foetal: Breathing of a foetus in the womb through the two channels of control and function of the microcosmic orbit ceasing to function when the umbilical cord is cut at birth and being replaced by breathing through the nostrils.

Breathing, Fourfold: A full fourfold breathing consists of in and out breaths with corresponding ascent and descent of inner fire in the microcosmic orbit which contributes to the immortal breath.

Breathing, Immortal: It rises in the heel pathway, from the heels to the brain and, descends in the trunk pathway, from the brain to the mortal gate. It is also called the self-winding wheel of the law, i.e. the macrocosmic orbit through which the vital breath goes up and down to restore the profound foetal breathing, thereby wiping out all postnatal conditions so that prenatal vitality can be transmuted into a bright pearl that illuminates the brain where an ambrosia produces and nurtures the immortal seed in the lower tan t'ien, in which it radiates, lighting up the heart heralding the formation of this immortal seed, when breathing appears to cease and the pulses seem to stop beating in the condition of complete serenity. See Self-winding wheel of the law.

Cardinal points of the microcosmic orbit, The four: 1. North (tzu) at the base of the penis, 2. South (wu), the top of the head, and, between them, 3. East (mao) on the back and 4. West (yu) in front of the body.

Cauldron: Cavity in which the process of alchemy transmutes the generative force into vitality and vitality into spirit. It changes place rising from the lower tan t'ien under the navel to the middle tan t'ien in the solar plexus to transmute the generative force into vitality, and then to the upper tan t'ien in the brain, called the precious cauldron, to transmute vitality into spirit.

Cavity of true vitality (chen ch'i hsueh): The lower tan t'ien under the navel where true vitality manifests. See Chen ch'i hsueh.

Cavity of vitality: The lower tan t'ien under the navel; also called Ocean of vitality (ch'i hai) and Gate to life (ming men).

Channel of control (tu mo): A psychic channel in the spine, from its base to the brain. It forms with the channel of function (jen mo) the microcosmic orbit.

Channel of function (jen mo): A channel in front of the body, from the brain to the base of the penis.

Chao Pi Ch'en: A Taoist master, born in 1860, who wrote the treatise Hsin Ming Fa Chueh Ming Chih or The Secrets of Cultivation of Essential Nature and Eternal Life, presented in this book.

Chen ch'i hsueh: Cavity of real vitality, or the lower tan t'ien 1·3 inches under the navel.

Chen hsi: True breath.

Chen hsin: True nature.

Chen jen: Immortal man.

Chiang kung: The solar plexus. See also Yellow hall (huang ting).

Ch'ien i: Heavenly oneness, a name given to the great emptiness by the Book of Change.

Chin lu: Golden stove, the lower tan t'ien one and one-third inches under the navel.

Chin tan: The golden elixir of immortality. See Golden elixir.

Chu: A weight equal to the twenty-fourth part of a tael which is the Chinese ounce, equal to one and one-third oz. avoirdupois.

Ch'un hsien: The genital duct which links the lower tan t'ien to the testicles, which the generative force reaches to change into semen.

Chun huo: Chief fire or heart's fire which is aroused by evil thoughts and should be avoided by the practiser.

Ch'ung mo: See The eight psychic channels.

Circle of light: A round light formed by spiritual vitality that springs from the middle tan t'ien or solar plexus after spirit and vitality have returned to the lower tan t'ien under the navel; it is the manifestation of the real nature of the self.

Cleansing and purifying (mu yu): *Cleansing* the positive ascent and *purifying* the negative descent during the microcosmic orbiting, for the positive is already pure and needs only some cleaning whereas the negative is corrupt and should be purified to be transmuted into the positive.

Coiling up the body into five dragons: A method which consists of 'composing' one's head (i.e. putting it in comfortable position), curving and reclining the body on either side, like the coiled length of a sleeping dragon or the curved body of a dog, bending one arm for a pillow while stretching the other to place a hand on the belly, and straightening one leg while bending the other. Even the heart is immersed in sleep, the pupils of both eyes should be drawn close to each other for pointed concentration on the great emptiness so that in the condition of utter stillness the vital principle returns automatically to its source (under the navel), breathing continues normally and so is self-regulated, and the (vital) breath is brought under perfect control. This method of sleeping will banish all dreams and so prevent the generative fluid from draining away.

Cold storage technique: Consists of driving the light of positive spirit manifesting in the brain into the lower abdomen with pointed concentration on vitality there until it vibrates. The practiser should then imagine that this vitality goes up and down in the thrusting channel between the heart and the lower abdomen until all of a sudden it slips into the lower tan t'ien; this is called *entry into the cavity within a cavity* and is actual *re-entry into the foetus for further creativity.*

Components, The four: Body, breath, incorporeal and corporeal souls symbolised by the elements of water, fire, wood and metal.

Copulation, Inner (nei chiao kou): By inner copulation of the positive and negative principles is meant the production of the microcosmic inner alchemical agent by rolling the eyes from left to right in conjunction with the passing of inner fire through sublimating phrases at the cardinal points D and J of the microcosmic orbit, for the purpose of transmuting vitality into spirit whose full development causes a bright light, called *the mysterious gate* (hsuan kuan) to manifest in the original cavity of spirit between and behind the eyes.

Creativity, Mechanism of: Way in which the process of creation works to transmute mortality into immortality, that is when the generative force, vitality and spirit unite to become one as shown by the circle of light in front of the practiser.

Divisions of One vitality, The two: The positive yang and negative yin as represented by the sun and the moon.

Dragon, The cavity of the: The lower tan t'ien cavity (see tan t'ien).

Dragon and Stork: Emblem of longevity.

Dragon and Tiger: Dragon stands for negative vitality and tiger for positive vitality. Their *copulation* brings into manifestation the original spirit in its bright light. See also Vitality, Positive and negative.

Dragon and tiger cavities: The negative and positive cavities in the centres of the left and right palms respectively.

Dragon's hum: Reveals the fullness of vitality in the generative force. When vitality fills the tiny channels of the nervous and psychic systems, it produces indistinct sounds.

Driving the three vehicles uphill: A technique which helps the macrocosmic alchemical agent to rise first slowly through the coccyx, the first gate at the base of the backbone, like a goat slowly drawing a cart up hill; then thrust through the second gate between the kidneys, like a deer speedily drawing a cart up hill; and finally to force through the occiput or third gate at the back of the head, like an ox drawing a cart up hill.

Earth: The lower abdomen.

Eating and sleeping: When the immortal seed matures the practiser does not want to sleep and when prenatal vitality is full he does not want to eat.

Elements, The five: Metal (chin), wood (mu), water (shui), fire (huo) and earth (t'u); the union of the five elements produces the elixir of immortality.

Elements, The three basic: The generative force, vitality and spirit. See also the Three precious elements and the Three treasures.

Elements, The three precious: The generative force, vitality and spirit. See also the Three Treasures and the Three Basic Elements.

Elixir of Immortality: Also called Golden Elixir; is produced by the union of generative force, vitality and spirit.

Emission, Involuntary: Wei hsien or risks at night.

Entry into the cavity within a cavity: Entry into the lower tan t'ien cavity within the lower abdomen (the house of water). See Cold Storage technique.

Eyes, Turning round the: There are three methods of turning round the eyes which have different purposes: a. macrocosmic sublimation of the *generative force* (see Chapter 4); b. microcosmic purification of *vitality* (see Chapter 6); and c. gathering prenatal basic vitality to invigorate *spirit* to produce the macrocosmic alchemical agent which develops when the light of vitality appears (see Chapter 7).

Families, The three (san chia): The body, heart and thought.

Feng fu: See Storehouse of the wind.

Field of Elixir (tan t'ien): The lower tan t'ien under the navel.

Fire, Quick and slow: Quick fire is produced by in and out breathing to put the vital force into orbit for purification; and slow fire is produced by a meditative method which consists of closing both eyes to develop a mind which, although void, does not cease to work, which, although radiant, does not continue to stay, and which is neither forgotten nor upheld. Quick fire shifts and slow fire calms, as the masters put it, and both transform impurities in the body into tears which are discharged through the eyes.

Fire, Spiritual: It produces the golden light which replaces a white light which has appeared in front of the practiser when his lower tan t'ien is full of the alchemical agent which reveals to his eyes the beauty of positive vital breath.

Fire used for purification has eighteen meanings:

(a) *Four kinds of fire kindled by breathing to transform the generative fluid derived from the digestion of food into generative force:*

1 Kindling the fire (to return the generative force to the lower tan t'ien)

2 Leading the fire (to turn the wheel of the law to gather the alchemical agent)

3 Forcing the fire with fire (i.e. breathing in and out to drive the generative and vital forces into the stove in the lower abdomen)

4 Stopping the fire (i.e. discontinuing all breathing after the golden light has manifested twice in order not to spoil the alchemical agent gathered).

(b) *Seven kinds of fire, derived from spirit, to transform the generative force into vitality:*

1 Freezing the fire (i.e. freezing and driving spirit into the lower tan t'ien)

2 Driving the fire (into) is driving into the microcosmic orbit the inner fire which then passes through the sublimating phases at D and J to gather the inner alchemical agent so that true vitality soars up to the brain which will then develop fully, causing a bright light, called the mysterious gate, to manifest between the eyes.

3 Lowering the fire (to cause the negative fire to retreat so that the positive yang develops fully and replaces the negative yin.)

4 Shifting the fire (is using quick fire to enlarge all obstructed channels to clear them of obstructions)-See Quick and slow fires.

5 Calming the fire (is using slow fire to help the psychic channels that have dilated to shrink so that the breath that has spread in the body can return to its former position under the navel) – See Quick and slow fires.

6 Fire in its own house is when the heart (the house of fire) is stirred and the penis stands erect in spite of the absence of thoughts; this is real fire in its house which arouses the genital organ and is not the genuine one which vibrates at the hour of tsu (11 p.m. to 1 a.m.) when the penis erects and when the alchemical agent should be gathered.

7 Heart's fire is the fire of passion excited by evil thoughts which arouse sexual desire; this is 'chief fire' (chun huo) or evil fire which should be avoided.

(c) *Seven kinds of fire derived from prenatal vitality, which purify the breathing and contribute to the manifestation of original spirit:*

1 Circulating the fire (up in the channel of control to the original cavity of spirit and down in the channel of function to the lower tan t'ien)

2 Gathering the fire is collecting the generative and vital forces as well as the alchemical agent to lift up the vital breath below in the twin cultivation of essential nature and eternal life.

3 Lifting the fire (which has been gathered to the brain before lowering it to the lower tan t'ien to invigorate the body

which has been weakened by the drain of generative force).

4 Fire in the house of water (k' an) stands for vitality in vibration which forms a bellows from below the heart to under the navel, which is linked with the genital gate through the mortal gate.

5 Negative fire in the stove or lower tan t'ien which drives vitality into the microcosmic orbit.

6 Fire immersed in water. When the generative and vital forces are in the lower tan t'ien they are fire in the house of water, but when they leave it to drain away they take a liquid form.

7 Fire in the stove. When spirit and vitality vibrate in the lower tan t'ien, this is fire in the stove.

Five dragons upholding the holy one (wu lung peng sheng): Five is the number of the element of earth which stands for the right thought; *dragon* stands for spirit, i.e. the practiser who is ready to sacrifice his body in his quest of immortality (by) *upholding the holy one* which means by looking up to suck up the ascending precious gem or the macrocosmic alchemical agent for the final breakthrough.

Five vital breaths: When the five vital breaths (in the heart, spleen, lungs, liver and kidneys) converge in the head, the golden light appears and unites with the white light of vitality which has manifested after the intermingling of the generative force, vitality and spirit. This is the union of the true positive and negative principles from which the immortal foetus emerges to take shape *Flute without holes (played in reverse):* The mechanism of breathing is closed (ho) so that outer air breathed in reaches the lower abdomen to push up the vital force in the channel of control to the brain, and is opened (p'i) to expel it from the lower abdomen while the vital force, now released from pressure, returns from the brain to the lower abdomen.

Foetus, Immortal (Tao foetus or True seed): The union of the white and golden lights produces the immortal foetus from which spirit will emerge to become immortal after the practiser, on seeing falling snow and dancing flowers, *stirs the thought* of leaping into the great emptiness. This thought will open the heavenly gate at the top of the head so that spirit can leave the physical body to appear in countless transformation bodies in space. (See immortal foetus.)

Foundation, Laying the (chu chi): When spirit wanders outside in quest of sense data, vitality dissipates and the generative force is corrupt. It is, therefore, necessary to sublimate the three precious elements, namely the generative force, vital breath and spirit to restore their original strength, and the foundation will be laid when these three elements unite leading to the formation of the immortal seed.

This foundation will lift the practiser from the mortal to the immortal plane, still his spirit within ten months, and enable him to give up sleep within nine or ten months, dispense with food and drink within ten months, feel neither cold in winter nor hot in summer, and achieve unperturbed spirit which leads to stable serenity.

This laying of the foundation will cause life to last as long as heaven and earth, and lead to the acquisition of the supernatural powers possessed by all immortals.

Four necessities for the practice of alchemy (on the mountain) : Utensils, money, companions and a suitable place for meditation. The utensils are: a round wooden object like a bun, covered with cotton, to sit on to block the anus; and a clothes-peg to close the nostrils. Money is to buy food for the practiser and his companions during the training.

Companions are friends also practising alchemy, to help him and pinch his backbone when required. The place is a quiet hut or temple not too far from towns and cities.

Freezing spirit: An alchemical process which ensures the condition of serenity in which the practiser becomes unconscious, his breathing almost ceases and his pulses seem to stop beating for the purpose of gathering prenatal true vitality in the original cavity of spirit in the centre of the brain and then driving it into the lower tan t'ien under the navel to hold it there to achieve immortal breathing. See Self-winding wheel of the law.

Gate to life (ming men): The lower tan t'ien which is below and behind the navel, and below and before the kidneys, the distance between it and the front and rear of the abdomen being in the proportion of seven to three. Also called the ocean or cavity of vitality. See Cavity of vitality and Ocean of vitality.

Generative force (ching): Essence of procreation which produces the generative fluid that satisfies sexual desire and begets offspring. *Genital organ, Retractile:* Which reveals the fullness of prenatal vitality in the body, a very good sign during the training in Taoist alchemy.

Gentle breeze (sun feng): Ventilation by in and out breathing. See Sun feng.

Golden elixir (chin tan): A radiant circle manifesting in the cavity of spirit between and behind the eyes. It stands for the supreme ultimate (t'ai chi) and the original awareness (yuan cheuh). See Elixir of immortality.

Golden light: Reveals the fullness of the luminous generative force, vitality and spirit.

Golden nectar: A liquid produced by the macrocosmic alchemical agent which has been successfully gathered by the practiser. When his mouth is full of this nectar he should swallow it with a gulp to drive it into the channel of function to the lower tan t'ien to seal vitality there. If he fails to gather the golden nectar he gets only pure saliva.

Hall of voidness (hsu shih) : The heart devoid of feelings and passions.

Hall, Yellow (huang ting): The middle tan t'ien in the solar plexus.

Heart: The house of fire and the organ of essential nature (hsin ken).

Heart and lower abdomen: The heart is the seat of fire (of passion) and the lower abdomen is the seat of water (of sexual pleasure). The fire above should be driven down into the water below, and the water below should be scorched by fire to become steam and be lifted to wipe out passion in order to achieve the stable equilibrium and harmony of fire and water. The heart and lower abdomen are respectively symbolised by the dragon (the female or negative vitality) and the tiger (the male or positive vitality).

Heart's fire (hsin huo): Or chief fire (chun huo) aroused by evil thoughts which should be avoided. See Chun huo.

Heaven and earth: The head and the abdomen.

Heavenly gate (miao men) : The aperture of Brahma at the top of the the head by which positive spirit comes out of the body.

Heavenly oneness (ch'ien i) : A name given to the great emptiness by the Book of Change. See Ch'ien i.

Heavenly palace (tzu fu): Another name of tsu ch'iao, the original cavity of spirit.

Heaventy pool (t'ien chih hsueh): A cavity in the palate by which vitality flows down to drain away. Hence the tongue is lifted up to plug it thereby making a bridge for vitality to come down through the hsuan ying cavity (the mysterious bridle) on the channel of function to the lower tan t'ien centre.

Heel and trunk pathways: The heel pathway (tung chung) from the heels to the brain and the trunk pathway (tung ti) from the brain to the trunk, i.e. the mortal gate. See Self-winding wheel of the law.

Ho and p'i: Ho is closing the mechanism of respiration while breathing in so that the air goes down to exert pressure on the lower abdomen causing the generative force to go up in the channel of control to the brain, and p'i is opening the mechanism of respiration while breathing out so that the air goes out of the body to relax pressure on the lower abdomen causing the generative force to descend in the channel of function from the brain to the lower abdomen.

Ho che: Microcosmic orbiting. See Water-wheels.

Horse of intellect, Running: See Monkey heart and running horse of intellect.

Hour of tsu: The beginning of the positive a.m. half of the day between 11 p.m. and 1 a.m. when the penis stands erect of itself in sleep in spite of the absence of thoughts and dreams. It is the proper moment to gather the generative force for sublimation, for the gathering of it during the negative p.m. half of the day is ineffective.

Houses of fire and water: Li, the heart, is the house of fire and k'an, the lower tan t'ien, is the house of water.

Hsiao yo: See Microcosmic outer alchemical agent.

Hsien t'ien and Hou t'ien: See Prenatal and postnatal.

Hsien t'ien chen chung: See Prenatal true seed.

Hsin hai: See Ocean of essential nature.

Hsin ken: The organ of essential nature. See Heart.

Hsin ming shuang hsiu: Cultivation of both essential nature and eternal life.

Hsu shih: The hall of voidness or the heart devoid of feelings and passions.

Hsuan chu: The real generative force. See Mysterious pearl.

Hsuan Ying: The *Mysterious bridle,* a cavity behind the *Heavenly pool* in the palate, by which vitality goes down in the channel of function in the microcosmic orbiting.

Huang Ting: The *Yellow hall* or middle tan t'ien in the solar plexus.

Huang Ya: Or *Yellow Bud:* The real generative force. See Yellow bud.

I kuan: The all-pervading one, a name given to the great emptiness by the Confucian classics.

Immaterial spirit (ch'ung ling): A minor channel linking the right side of the original cavity of spirit with the heavenly valley (tien ku) above it and the yung chuan (bubbling spring) centre in the centre of the right foot after running through the heart in the chest.

Immersion of fire in water: Concentration on the lower tan t'ien to direct the element of fire in the heart to scorch the element of water in the lower abdomen, thus emptying the heart of passion and stopping water in the lower abdomen from flowing down in order to achieve the stable equilibrium of water and fire. See Shui huo chi chi.

Immortal foetus (tao foetus or true seed): An incorporeal manifestation of the union of vitality and spirit as shown by the union of the white and golden lights. It has neither form nor shape and is unlike any ordinary foetus, the outcome of sexual intercourse.

Immortal seed: The crystallisation of positive generative force the fullness of which manifests as the white light of vitality while the fullness of the immortal seed manifests as a golden light which reveals the negative vitality within the generative force. The light of the eyes directed downward is positive and when the positive and negative lights meet, a precious light (pao kuang) will emerge. See Immortal foetus.

The six signs of the formation of the immortal seed are: 1. a golden light appearing in the eyes; 2. the back of the head vibrates audibly; 3. the dragon's hum is heard in the right and 4. the tiger's roar in the left ear; 5. fire blazes in the lower tan t'ien, bubbles rise in the body, spasms shake the nose, and 6. the genital organ draws in.

Immortals: Earth-bound immortals (shen hsien) and heavenly immortals (chin hsien).

Jen mo: See Channel of function and Psychic channels, the eight.

K'an: The house of water in the lower abdomen (See K'an and li).

K'an and li: The lower abdomen and the heart respectively. Spirit in li (the house of fire) is essential nature, and vitality in k'an (the house of water) is eternal life.

Kan lu: See Sweet dew.

Keeping vigil over a dead body: When spirit fails to come out of the foetus after the practiser has seen falling snow and dancing flowers, this is called *keeping vigil over a dead body.* This is caused by the practiser who takes delight in the state of serenity thereby forgetting about leaving the foetus.

Kun huo: Negative fire in the stove, i.e. the lower tan t'ien.

Lao Tsu: Born in 604 B.C. Named Li Erh, and also called Li Po Yang, he was a native of K'u district in Ch'u state (now Hupeh province). He was for a long time a censor under the Chou dynasty, but seeing that it began to decline he left the country for an unknown destination. At the request of the official defending the pass at the frontier he wrote the Tao Te Ching. According to the legend then current, he was already old at birth, hence he was called Lao Tsu or 'Old Son'.

Lao Tsu was determined to revive the ancient tradition prevalent at the time of emperor Huang Ti (2698-2597 B.C.). Since Huang Ti was the founder of Taoism which Lao Tsu later revived it is called the doctrine of Huang-Lao.

Lead: A Taoist technical term which means vitality or the vital principle.

Li: The heart or house of fire (of passions). See K'an and li.

Life, Cavity of (ming ch'iao): The lower tan t'ien under the navel.

Life, Eternal: Endless life of an immortal man, the aim of Taoist alchemy.

Light, White and Golden (Hui kuang and shan kuang): When the generative force has been purified and fully developed, it rises to the brain to unite with essential nature, causing the *white light* of vitality to manifest like moonlight; and when vitality is full and descends to the lower tan t'ien to unite with eternal life, the *golden light* of the immortal seed manifests. The union of these two lights produces the immortal foetus which then returns to the original cavity of spirit in the brain for the final breakthrough.

Lower abdomen: The house of water as contrasted with the heart which is the house of fire. The lower abdomen is frequently referred to as the lower tan t'ien cavity under the navel.

Lower tan t'ien: See Tan t'ien.

Lung Kung: The cavity of the dragon, which is the lower tan t'ien cavity. See Tan t'ien.

Magpie bridge: The upper magpie bridge (shang ch'ueh ch'iao) is the nasal duct; the middle magpie bridge (chung ch'ueh ch'iao) is the tongue; and the lower magpie bridge (hsia ch'ueh ch'iao) is the anus.

Male and female principle: The male (chien) or positive and the female (k'un) or negative principle.

Mercury: A Taoist technical term meaning spirit.

Miao men: The aperture of Brahma on the top of the head. See Heavenly gate.

Microcosmic orbit (Hsiao chou tien): It begins at the base of the spine, called the first gate (wei lu), rising in the backbone to the second gate between the kidneys (chia chi) and then to the back of the head, called the third gate (yu ch'en), before reaching the brain, to descend down the face, chest and abdomen to return to where it rose and so completes a full circuit.

Microcosmic orbit, The six phases of the (liu hou) : Rising in the channel of control from the mortal gate A to D and G at the top of the head (see *figure 2)* are the first, second and third positions in the ascent, and sinking in the channel of function from G to J and A which are the first, second and third positions in the descent.

Microcosmic orbit, The two phases of the (chin yang tui yin): Ascent of positive fire (chin yang) in the channel of control and descent of negative fire (tui yin) in the channel of function.

Middle tan t'ien: See Tan t'ien.

Ming ch'iao: See Cavity of life.

Ming men: See Gate to life.

Monkey heart and running horse of intellect: When one breathes in and out, one's concentration causes the generative force to rise and fall in the microcosmic orbit thus slowly turning the wheel of the law. By counting from one to ten and then from ten to one hundred breaths, with the mind following the counting to prevent it from wandering outside, the mind and the counting will be in unison; this is called *locking up the monkey heart and tying up the running horse of intellect.*

Moon: The right eye which stands for the negative yin. It also stands for the lower tan t'ien under the navel.

Mortal gate (sheng szu ch'iao): The base of the penis by which the generative fluid drains away.

Mysterious gate (Hsuan kuan): The bright light which manifests when spirit is fully developed for the breakthrough, i.e. the mysterious entrance to immortality.

Mysterious pearl (Hsuan chu): The real generative force. See Hsuan chu.

Nature, Essential: Man's real nature which is undying, the realisation of which is the aim of Taoist alchemy.

Nature, Ocean of essential (hsin hai): Also called tsu ch'iao or the original cavity of spirit between and behind the eyes.

Nature, True: Prenatal vitality in its cell (ch'i pao) on the top of the medulla oblongata.

Negative embracing the positive, The: See Positive embracing the negative and vice versa.

Nei chiao kou: See Inner copulation.

Ni wan: Literally 'Ball of mud' i.e. the brain or region of the brain. Frequently referred to as the original cavity of spirit between and behind the eyes, like the lower belly which is usually mentioned as the lower tan t'ien about one and a half inches under the navel.

Nine unsettled breaths, The: Caused by anger which lifts and fear which lowers the breath; by joy which slows it down; by grief which disperses it; by terror which throws it out of gear; by thinking which ties it up; by toil which wastes it; by cold which collects and heat which scatters it.

Northern sea: The lower tan t'ien cavity. See Tan t'ien.

Obliterating meditation: Or extinguishing meditation, i.e. meditation which wipes out all traces of the worldly.

Ocean of vitality: The lower tan t'ien cavity under the navel. See Tan t'ien.

Original awareness (yuan chueh): See Golden elixir.

Original cavity of spirit: (Yuan Shen Shih or tsu ch'iao, the ancestral cavity) a spot between and behind the eyes, where a light manifests when the practiser succeeds in concentrating on it.

Pai hui: See Source of the nervous system.

P'i: See Ho and p'i.

Pi kuan, K'ai kuan: Chinese terms which mean shutting and opening the mysterious gate by rolling the eyes thirty-six times to follow the four phases of microcosmic sublimation of vitality ascending from cardinal point A to D, G and J, and twenty-four times to follow it descending from G to D, A and J.

Poles, The four: Prenatal heaven and earth and postnatal heart and abdomen.

Positive and negative fires: During the microcosmic orbiting the fire that goes up in the channel of control to the brain is positive fire (yang huo) and the fire that goes down in the channel of function is negative fire (yin fu).

Positive (yang) embracing the negative (yin) and vice versa, The: In the meditation posture, when the left leg is placed outside and close to the right one, this is the positive embracing the negative; and when the thumb of the left hand touches its middle finger and the right hand is placed under it (palm upward) with its thumb bent over the left palm, this is the negative embracing the positive. This is to form a circuit of eight psychic channels, and is also the linking of the four limbs to shut the four gates so that the centre can be held on to.

Positive fire, The three manifestations of: When the golden light appears for the first time the practiser should obtain the four necessities for advanced training, i.e. utensils, money, companion and a suitable place for meditation to maintain the union of the lights of essential nature and eternal life. As time passes the golden light will suddenly reappear much brighter; this is the second manifestation of positive light. He should now stop the fire to gather the macrocosmic alchemical agent. To stop fire is to cease regulating his breathing and circulating vital air which should be replaced by the heart, spirit and thought combined to go up in the channel of control and down in the channel of function. When this golden light appears for the third time he should immediately grasp the macrocosmic alchemical agent for the breakthrough in order to transmute vitality into spirit thereby leaping over the worldly to the divine state. The fourth manifestation of the golden light will reveal the practiser's failure to stop the fire by his wrong use of in and out breaths at this stage, for the macrocosmic agent will follow that fire to drain away in the form of postnatal generative fluid, thereby nullifying all progress so far achieved.

Positive generative force (yang ching): The real generative force See Yang ching.

Prenatal (hsien t'ien) and postnatal (hou t'ien): 'Prenatal' denotes the positive or spiritual nature originally existing before birth and 'postnatal' means its negative or corrupt counterpart which follows the ordinary way of material life after birth, the former being real and permanent whereas the latter is illusory and transient.

Prenatal true seed (hsien t'ien chen chung): The union of spirit and vitality into one single gem.

Psychic centre, cavity, cell, abode, seat, house, etc.: These technical terms are used in Taoist texts and the duty of a translator is not to change them. When vitality develops and pervades every part in the body the practiser feels as if countless tiny fishes are swimming in his body and limbs to enter the muscles, nerves, bones and marrows, filling all hollows, pockets, holes, dents, depressions, interstices, etc. which then take various forms and shapes as Chuang Tzu

describes the effects of the 'wind' which causes huge trees to
have hollows and openings like noses, mouths, ears, jugs,
cups, mortars, etc. Only those who have succeeded in
transmuting the generative force into vitality have this
unusual experience and understand what Chuang Tzu
means, and also why the ancients used more than one single
term in the texts.

This note is added because we have been asked why we have
not used one technical term that is either 'centre' or the
Hindu word 'cakra' throughout this volume.

Psychic channels, The eight (ch'i ching pa mo) : The eight main
psychic channels:

1 The channel of control (tu mo) rises from the base of the
penis and passes through the coccyx up the backbone to the
brain;

2 The channel of function (jen mo) rises from the base of
the penis and goes up along the belly, passes through the
navel, the pit of the stomach, the chest and throat, up to the
brain;

3 The belt channel (tai mo) from both sides of the navel
forming a belt which circles the belly;

4 The thrusting channel (ch'ung mo) rises from the base of
the penis, goes up between the tu mo and jen mo channels
and ends in the heart;

5 The positive arm channels (yang yu) in the outer sides of
both arms, link both shoulders with the centres of the palms
after passing through the middle fingers;

6 The negative arm channels (yin yu) in the inner sides of
both arms, link the centres of the palms with the chest;

7 The positive leg channels (yang chiao) rise from the
centres of the soles and turn along the outer sides of the

ankles and legs before reaching the base of the penis where
they connect with other channels;

8 The negative leg channels (yin chiao) rise from the centres
of the soles and turn along the inner sides of the ankles and
legs before reaching the base of the penis where they connect
with other channels.

Purifying: See Cleaning and purifying.

Re-entry into the foetus for further creativity: The outcome of
the entry into a foetus is the birth of a man into the world,
and his subsequent practice of Taoist alchemy causes him to
re-enter a spiritual foetus to become an immortal.

Returning a myriad things to one whole: In order to develop the
immortal foetus fully the practiser should concentrate on
spirit forgetting all about the foetus which is within his spirit.
This is called 'returning a myriad things to one whole'.

Seed, The true: See Immortal foetus.

Serenity: Minor serenity (hsiao ting ching) lasts only one day
in which dullness and confusion cause the practiser to be
unconscious, like a dying man who is breathless; medium
serenity (chung ting ching) lasts three successive days; and
major serenity (ta ting ching) seven successive days.

Serenity, The four stages of: Thoughtlessness (nien chu),
breathlessness (hsi chu), pulselessness (mo chu) and
extinction (unmindfulness) of worldly existence (mieh chin).

Seven passions that damage vitality, The: Intense delight that
harms the heart; intense anger the liver; grief the lungs; fear
the gall bladder; love spirit; hate the disposition; and intense
desire the stomach.

Sheng szu ch'iao: The mortal gate at the base of the penis, by which the generative fluid is discharged.

Shou i: Holding on to one i.e. the great emptiness.

Shui huo chi chi: Water and fire in equilibrium. When fire is immersed in water it stops soaring up thereby causing the heart to be empty, and when water is scorched by fire it becomes steam and stops flowing down. This is water and fire in stable equilibrium which will in time produce true vitality. See Immersion of fire in water.

Six transcendental powers: To realise: 1 stoppage of all drain of the generative and vital forces; 2 divine sight; 3. divine hearing; 4. knowledge of past lives; 5. understanding of other minds; and 6. divine mirror.

Snow and flowers: When the immortal foetus is fully developed snow and flowers are seen falling in disorder by the practiser.

Solar plexus: The middle tan t'ien; also called Chiang kung and Huang ting.

Source of the nervous system: Pai hui literally 'the point where *hundreds meet*' on the top of the head.

Spirit (shen): The divine in man or his immortal nature which derives from the purification of vitality. Spirit leads to the realisation of essential nature and vitality to eternal life which are the aim of Taoist alchemy.

Spirit, Positive and negative: The negative spirit (yin shen), visible to the practiser when he closes his eyes, is created by the first five of six transcendental powers, and is the negative spiritual breath which can see others but is invisible to them, cannot speak to them and cannot pick up objects, and is, therefore, mortal in the end. The positive spirit (yang shen) is created by the five kinds of eyes and six transcendental powers, is visible to others, can speak to them, can pick up objects and has the same features of the practiser's own body. It takes form when it gathers in one place, or becomes pure vitality when it scatters to fill the great emptiness which will be its boundless body. See Six transcendental powers.

The five kinds of eye are: the heavenly eye which sees all things in the thirty-three heavens; the earthly eye which sees the eighteen hells; the spiritual eye, or eye of vitality, which sees past and future events in the world; the human eye which sees happenings before birth and death; and the ghostly eye which sees through the mountains, earth and metals.

Spirit-vitality: After spirit and vitality have returned to the lower tan t'ien under the navel, their union, called spirit-vitality, produces the spiritual light which springs from the middle tan t'ien or solar plexus.

Stirring the thought of jumping into the great emptiness: To open the heavenly gate on the top of the head in order to leap into the great emptiness otherwise the practiser will fail to emerge from the immortal foetus.

Storehouse of the wind (feng fu) : A cavity of the element of the wind in the back of the head.

Stove (lu): A cavity where the inner fire is kindled by regulated breathing to put the generative force into microcosmic orbit and transmute it into vitality. The stove remains in the lower tan t'ien cavity throughout the process of alchemy.

Suck: Drawing nourishment from the body.

Sucking (hsi), pressing (shih), pinching (ts'o) and shutting (pi), The method of: To gather the macrocosmic alchemical agent and help its ascent in the channel of control by *shutting* the anus with a wooden bun, by *pressing* the tongue against the palate and a finger on the mortal gate, by *sucking* in a breath through the nose and by *pinching* the backbone above the coccyx to warm and loosen the marrow at the base of the spine.

Sun: The left eye which stands for the positive yang; it also stands for the heart.

Sun and moon: The two eyes.

Sun and moon, The union of the: When the pupils of both eyes are drawn close to each other in a squint for pointed concentration so that the heart (fire) and lower abdomen (water) are linked for the production of prenatal vitality.

Sun feng: Gentle breeze or ventilation by in and out breathing.

Supreme Ultimate (tai chi): The circle of tai chi wherein real positive vitality and essential nature unite to emit the light of vitality which is the light of true nature in the precious cauldron in the brain and that of true life in the stove in the lower abdomen. See Golden elixir.

Sweet dew (kan lu): Pure saliva. See Ambrosia.

Symbols, The four (szu hsiang): Prenatal heaven and earth and postnatal heart and abdomen gathered in the solar plexus to produce the macrocosmic alchemical agent.

Szu ko yin yang: See the four yin-yang.

Ta ting: Utter serenity.

Tai chi: See supreme ultimate and Golden elixir.

Tai Mo: The belt channel. See the eight psychic channels.

Tan t'ien: Lit. 'field of the drug' i.e. a psychic centre where the drug or alchemical agent is produced. There are three tan t'ien in the body: 1. the lower tan t'ien, about one and a half inches under the navel where the generative force is retained so that it does not slip down and drain away, in order to purify it; 2. the middle tan t'ien, or the solar plexus, where the generative force is transmuted into vitality; and 3. the upper tan t'ien or the original cavity of spirit between and behind the eyes, where vitality is transmuted into spirit. The lower tan t'ien is also called the cavity or ocean of vitality, lung kung or the cavity of the dragon, and northern sea.

Tao: Prenatal spirit-vitality; the union of essential nature and eternal life, spirit being essential nature and vitality being eternal life.

Tao foetus: The immortal foetus. See Immortal foetus.

Ten excesses that injure vitality, The: Excessive walking that harms the nerves; standing the bones; sitting the blood; sleep the pulses; joy the generative force; looking (at things) spirit; speaking the breath; thinking the stomach; eating the heart; and too much sex the life.

Threefold continual ascension (san ch'ien fa): The generative force, vitality and spirit united into a bright moonlight which rises from the lower to the middle and then to the upper tan t'ien before the practiser sees falling snow and dancing flowers in front of him.

T'ien hsien: A heavenly immortal.

Tiger: See Dragon and tiger.

Tiger's roar: The sound of fully developed vitality which is active.

T'o yo: See Bellows.

Treasures, The three (san pao): Or three Basic elements (san yuan) are: the generative force, vitality and spirit. See also The three precious elements and the three basic elements.

Trunk pathway: See Heel and trunk pathways.

Ts'ai ch'u: Gathering the generative force for sublimation.

Tu mo: The channel of control. See the Channel of control and the Eight psychic channels.

Tung chung and tung ti: See Heels and trunk pathways.

Tzu fu: Heavenly palace, another name of tsu ch'iao, the original cavity of spirit. See Heavenly palace.

Umbilial cord: Before the umbilical cord is cut the baby's essential nature and eternal life are inseparable; this state is called prenatal. At birth his body becomes mortal because of the postnatal conditions of nature and life which are no longer united but divided into two, and so become unconnected.

Upper tan t'ien: See Tan t'ien.

Vital breaths, The five: These come from the vitality in the lower tan t'ien cavity from which they spread to the five viscera: to the lungs as the vital breath of the element of metal; to the heart as the vital breath of the element of fire; to the liver as the vital breath of the element of wood; to the stomach as the vital breath of the element of earth; and to the lower abdomen as the vital breath of the element of water. Their union into one vitality causes the golden light to manifest.

Vitality (ch'i): The vital principle derived from the purification of the generative force; it stands for eternal life.

Vitalities of nature and life: Nature-vitality is negative and life-vitality is positive; their union produces the true seed of immortality which will become the immortal foetus. The light of nature-vitality is like moonlight and the light of life-vitality is golden.

Vitality, Positive and negative: Positive vitality is male vitality that soars up and negative vitality is female vitality that goes down. They are symbolised by the tiger and dragon respectively. See Dragon and Tiger.

Vitality, Prenatal one true: Real vitality existing in the original cavity of spirit between and behind the eyes as revealed by the circle of light which Confucius called 'virtuous perfection (jen)', the Book of Change calls the 'Ultimateless (wu chi)', the Buddha 'perfect knowledge (yuan ming)' and the Taoists the 'elixir of immortality or spiritual light'.

Voidness: Voidness that is relative and empty does not radiate whereas voidness that is absolute and is not empty is spiritual light which is spirit-vitality that springs from the middle tan t'ian in the solar plexus.

Water-wheels (ho che): The microcosmic orbiting.

Wheel of the law (fa lun): The microcosmic orbiting caused by in and out breathing.

Wheel of the law, Self-winding: Automatic immortal breathing caused by the rise of postnatal vital breath from the heels to soar in the channel of control to the brain and its fall in the channel of function from the brain to the trunk or mortal gate, which, if continued for some time, will vibrate prenatal true vitality in the lower tan t'ien causing the latter to rise also in the channel of control and descend in the channel of function. These ascents and descents of postnatal breath, followed by those of prenatal true vitality, will result in automatic immortal breathing, called the self-winding wheel of the law. See Immortal breathing.

Wu chi: The ultimateless.

Yang: The positive, male, active, advance, progression.

Yang ch'iao: See The Eight psychic channels.

Yang ching: Real positive generative force. See Positive generative force.

Yang kuan: The genital gate, the opening at the end of the penis.

Yang yu: See The Eight psychic channels.

Yellow bud: The real generative force. See Huang Ya.

Yin: The negative, female, passive, retreat, retrogression.

Yin-yang, The four: The prenatal heaven and earth and postnatal heart and abdomen are called the four yin-yang (Szu ko yin yang), i.e. the four positive and negative principles.

Yin ch'iao: See The Eight psychic channels.

Yuan chueh: Original awareness. See Golden elixir.

Yinyu: See The Eight psychic channels.

INDEX